BY MARK LAUREN

You Are Your Own Gym
Body by You
Body Fuel

BODY FUEL

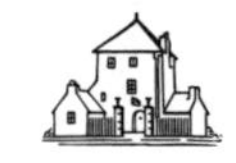

BALLANTINE BOOKS

NEW YORK

BODY FUEL

CALORIE-CYCLE YOUR WAY TO REDUCED BODY FAT AND GREATER MUSCLE DEFINITION

MARK LAUREN

WITH MAGGIE GREENWOOD-ROBINSON

Body Fuel proposes a program of diet and exercise recommendations for the reader to follow. However, you should consult a qualified medical professional (and, if you are pregnant, your ob-gyn) before starting this or any other fitness program. As with any diet or exercise program, if at any time you experience discomfort, stop immediately and consult your physician.

A Ballantine Books Trade Paperback Original

Published in the United States by Ballantine Books,
an imprint of Random House, a division of
Penguin Random House LLC, New York.

BALLANTINE and the HOUSE colophon are registered
trademarks of Penguin Random House LLC.

Photography by Timon Haringa

LIBRARY OF CONGRESS CATALOGING-IN-PUBLICATION DATA
Names: Lauren, Mark, author. | Greenwood-Robinson, Maggie, author.
Title: Body fuel: calorie-cycle your way to reduced body fat and greater muscle definition / Mark Lauren, Maggie Greenwood-Robinson.
Description: New York: Ballantine Books, 2016. | Includes bibliographical references.
Identifiers: LCCN 2015035980 | ISBN 9780553394955 (paperback: acid-free paper) | ISBN 9780553394962 (ebook)
Subjects: LCSH: Weight loss—Popular works. | Physical fitness—Popular works. | Nutrition—Popular works. | Metabolism—Popular works. | Reducing diets—Recipes. | BISAC: HEALTH & FITNESS / Nutrition. | HEALTH & FITNESS / Exercise. | HEALTH & FITNESS / General.
Classification: LCC RM222.2 .L357 2016 | DDC 641.5/638—dc23
LC record available at http://lccn.loc.gov/2015035980

Printed in the United States of America on acid-free paper

randomhousebooks.com

9 8 7 6 5 4 3 2 1

Book design by Mary A. Wirth

Contents

PART 4. THE BODY FUEL WORKOUT

Introduction

FUELING FAT LOSS

My nutritional philosophy stems from my military background as a Special Ops trainer. For eleven years, I was responsible for preparing hundreds of trainees for the extreme demands of serving in the U.S. Special Operations community. These trainees had to get lean and strong in record time, since the likelihood of survival and mission success would largely depend on their physical fitness.

My mode of physical training involved exercises based solely on using the resistance of a person's body weight—all done without the need for a posh state-of-the-art fitness facility. Using the "gym" of their bodies, soldiers were able to train themselves to be quick, agile, and powerful. This training method was tougher and more grueling than any workout using equipment, trust me. Once in combat, these soldiers could run fast, jump, push, roll, stop and start, change direction, get up or down, move under fire, and do other crucial warfare skills—in split seconds. If they were deficient in any of these fitness parameters, their chances of compromising the mission or becoming a liability to the team rose dramatically.

To fuel that type of live-or-die performance, my trainees had to eat for energy, strength, and physique perfection. Nutrition could not be overlooked; I had to develop and teach a diet that would deliver those benefits. The food had to be wholesome, natural, and pure. Look at it this way: if you saw someone build a hurricane shelter out of wood that was rotted or bricks that were broken, you'd know that the building would not have structural integrity and you wouldn't (shouldn't!) trust it to withstand hurricane-force winds.

The same is true of the nutritional building blocks you require to nourish and fuel your body. These building blocks include lean protein, natural carbohydrates, healthful fats, vitamins, minerals, and water—basically everything you eat and drink in order to construct a strong, vibrant, physically fit body.

So, to my way of thinking, the one "perfect" diet was similar to what cave-dwelling humans ate, except with the flexibility to use more recent food sources to maximize the benefits of intense training. After all, my trainees went through frequent, prolonged periods of highly intense activity, and their level of physical exertion was often as high as or higher than that of ancient hunters and gatherers. To get the absolute most out of my previously soft, untrained trainees, I had to develop an easy-to-follow, customizable nutritional plan based on natural, whole foods and plenty of protein.

Like my bestselling exercise books, *You Are Your Own Gym* and *Body by You,* the Body Fuel plan was thus born out of necessity—the need to help create and then maintain lean, physically capable human beings in record time.

In people who followed it, the results were obvious: Stored body fat burned efficiently. Energy levels were through the roof. Muscles became well developed and chiseled.

The diet turned out to be simple, too, the foods easy to remember—no illogical nutritional frills, just like my no-frills exercise program. This is a diet you can do anywhere, as you can my workout. Both are portable and easy—just what we need in today's busy, overscheduled world—and thus scalable to anyone's lifestyle, whether you are a regular civilian or a trainee fighting to stay in one of the most mentally and physically demanding programs in the world.

Just because I developed this way of eating to fuel bodies under extreme pressure to get and stay in tip-top shape, you shouldn't think for a moment that this diet is extreme. And it's not exclusionary. It lets you eat carbs. It lets you eat fat. It lets you eat all sorts of foods otherwise banned on most diets.

With these allowances, you'll drop body fat, recontour yourself with lean muscle, and improve your performance. Day by day on this plan, your body becomes accustomed to burning more fuel from stored body fat, because you'll be manipulating the quality and quantity of your calories and maximizing your natural fat-burning capacity.

The result: a defined, sculpted, and athletic body.

The food on this plan comes from *real fuel*, those foods closest to what our ancient ancestors ate, including meats, fish, vegetables, fruit, grains, nuts, and seeds—essentially natural, power-packed food, put together in a diet that is most compatible with our genetic makeup. Millions of years ago, people who ate these foods and used them to fuel their physically demanding lives were the fittest of the species, the survivors. Eating whole foods, close to the way they're found in nature, is the reason we can perform at our best—and look our best.

FOOD IS FUEL

In addition to training military Special Ops personnel, I have personally trained many civilians directly and hundreds of thousands of men and women around the world through my books, DVDs, and digital media. The feedback from these people, whose body type may not be of life-or-death importance but who nonetheless want to get in tip-top shape, has been largely the same—the long-term relationship with body fat is that they want to get rid of it and it wants to stay. In fact, the best way to describe its behavior would be resolute, clingy, and stubborn. I'm sure many of you are fighting the same battle. Which is why one in two Americans is now overweight, one in five is obese, and the ratio is even higher at all-you-can-eat buffets.

A lot of people these days are trying to excuse their weight problem by blaming it on their genes. That makes some sense to me, though I resist the idea that our genes are the number one culprits because we have basically the same genes today that our trimmer, fitter grandparents and great-grandparents had. What's changed is our lifestyles—more lazing around eating junk food, less moving around from exercise and daily activities. If you're frustrated with your weight, don't just blame your genes and let yourself get bigger and bigger. Do something about it. I'm here to help you.

One of the first things you can do, this very instant, is change your mind-set toward food. Think of food as fuel. What you eat should empower you. The main purpose of food is to nourish and provide you with a steady source of energy to take on your daily challenges. Truth is, I like fried chicken and apple pie as much as the next person, but a baked chicken breast and a juicy apple fill me up just as well, and without the added fat and sugar of the less nutritional preparations, they are good fuels that make you strong and healthy.

Not only will giving your body the right fuel change your looks for the better, but it will change your sex drive, skin, mood, energy, stress levels, mental and physical performance, and overall health. Every single cell of your body is affected by how you choose to fuel your body.

Once you adopt the mind-set that "food is fuel" and live by that motto, the results will blow you away. You'll find there is nothing you can't do.

A PREVIEW OF COMING ATTRACTIONS

Like a movie trailer that shows all the good parts with fast-paced editing—*whirl, punch, zow*—here's a preview of how *Body Fuel* plays out.

Fueling your body on my plan involves understanding some important distinctions about carbs. I categorize them as slow-fuel carbs or fast-fuel carbs, based on how they affect your blood sugar, energy levels, and fat-burning ability. Knowing when to reach for slow- or fast-fuel carbs, and how to balance them with protein and fat fuels, will help you optimize your results so that you experience only the steady loss of pounds and inches, week after week, while getting the absolute most out of your physical activities. Chapters 1 and 2 will help you master what you need to know about these important nutritional building blocks.

Once you understand the basics of the actual fuel you'll be eating, Chapter 3 will explain my innovative way you'll be building meals on this plan: "calorie cycling," periodically moving your calories down for a week or two by reducing the number of fast-fuel carbs that you consume. Calorie cycling is a "secret weapon" in the Body Fuel plan. This is how you're going to trick your metabolism into working at its hardest for you now and long into the future. Understand this simple three-tier approach to building your meals and you'll have the tool at hand to combat weight loss plateaus and weight gain for life. By changing the amount of calories you take in, you recharge your metabolism—a process that naturally leads to more body-firming muscle and less unsightly fat than if you were to follow a calorie-steady regimen for weeks on end. If you're like most of the people I train and advise, I think you'll love the concept of following a program that allows you to understand how fast-fuel carbs affect your performance and body composition, so you can customize your plan to *your* exact needs, while regularly changing up your food plan. Here's how you'll do it.

The Body Fuel diet consists of three eating "blocks," each with differing amounts of carbs and calories. This system is easy to remember and easy to incorporate into any lifestyle, but the most important thing is that cycling through the blocks is something you can customize and keep doing and doing and doing. You can eat this way for the rest of your life. Your body and metabolism won't become accustomed to the same old eating patterns—which lead to weight loss plateaus or ruts—but instead will continuously be tricked and triggered so that you continue to burn fuel efficiently and stay lean and strong, even after you've reached your goal weight or clothing size. Same blocks, but a fooled body every time.

The first block is the most liberal phase of the diet, and happily for you, it lasts the longest: three weeks (or even longer if you're making good progress on it), which is why I call it Block 3. You can have a lot of the fast-fuel carbs you love—one serving at each meal and one snack, for a total of four carbs daily. Think bread, pasta, potatoes, rice, and all sorts of fruit. Can you believe it? Don't worry: you can lose a chunk of weight by eating these fuels. And you won't even feel like you're dieting. It's a dream: the return of good food, which is absolutely necessary in the right doses for the development of an athletic, fat-burning body.

After three or more weeks of that, you'll be noticeably more energetic and trimmer. The scale will register a big drop in weight. The mirror will show a fitter you. Your clothes will fit better; in fact, you may have to go shopping for a smaller size. And you'll feel more energetic, simply by making realistic, sustainable, and important dietary changes.

Block 2 comes next and, you guessed it, lasts two weeks. During this block, you'll continue to eat most of the same foods, but with one exception: you'll reduce your carbs slightly, to two fast-fuel carbs a day. This way of eating initiates calorie cycling, explained briefly above. Overall, Block 2 is a little less liberal than Block 3, food-wise, but it keeps you in a fat-burning mode so you can taper down to your ideal weight.

Block 1 lasts for one week and is the most restrictive of the blocks. But remember, it's only one week, and then you go back to the top with Block 3 to eat more liberally. In Block 1 you'll cut your carbs down to one carb a day. Don't panic: anyone can do anything if it's just for seven days. You'll be amazed at how well you'll breeze through this week. The weight loss you've experienced up to this point will motivate you to tighten up your food choices, and you won't miss those extra carbs one bit. Even if you find Block 1 easy, it's important to cycle back to the eating style of Block 3 thereafter, especially if you're engaged in intense physical activity.

I don't want to give away the entire plot of the diet here, but let me emphasize that using these blocks is the key to looking and feeling your best through proper nutrition. You'll love this way of eating, because you're always changing up your diet and discovering how to adjust your food intake to get the results you want. You'll never get bored. You'll never be scratching your head about what to eat, because I lay it all out for you in simple terms. And you'll advance your knowledge about what and when to eat, so the diet becomes second nature to you. This will be the plan you use for the rest of your life.

A FAIL-SAFE PLAN

Fail-safe is a term normally used in the military to describe an operation designed to work or function automatically to prevent a breakdown or system failure. That's what the Body Fuel plan provides you with. Most diets fail because they are extreme and just don't fit into real life. For instance, if you have a diet plan that excludes a certain food—say pasta—and you go to an Italian restaurant, you can't have the most prominent (and probably best-prepared) thing on the menu, and that will elicit some frustration. Frustration builds on frustration, and before you know it, you're eating not only pasta but also everything else that's forbidden. When you overrestrict food, you set yourself up to possibly binge on everything you supposedly can't have. Your weight comes back, with interest.

Food deprivation is the last thing you want if you're looking to knock off pounds. There's even a psychological backlash, because when you binge on "forbidden" foods, you go on a guilt trip afterward. This is damaging to your psyche, makes you feel bad about yourself, and might even make you lose faith in your ability to get in shape—in short, a real downer. You're better than that! Once you know you can eat a wider range of foods on the Body Fuel plan—a key fail-safe characteristic of the diet—you won't have to wrangle with forbidden foods, and you'll lose the mental misery of feeling out of control.

Most diets fail because they leave you hungry; they just don't let you eat *enough*, or they banish some key element of a healthful diet. With the varied selection of foods and food combinations on Body Fuel, it's very unlikely that you'll get hungry. In fact, you'll feel energized. No more negative mood swings, either, because you'll be stabilizing your blood glucose levels, while getting *all* the nutrients you need.

Not only has extreme dieting been shown to set you up for failure, but it also slows your metabolism, making it very difficult to lose body fat and even easier to gain it. A slow metabolism can also make it hard to keep weight off in the future. Even if these diets work initially, it's highly unlikely that they'll work for long, because as we advance our fitness, our "margin of error" decreases, meaning that we need the flexibility to customize our diet (and exercise program) in order to continue progressing. In other words, at the start, any sort of restrictive diet will work; the true test is in a diet's ability to keep you moving forward after the first couple of months. For the long term, you need a flexible plan.

ONE MORE CLIP

Body Fuel, with its easy-to-remember food choices and meal combinations, is a highly effective way to lose body fat and gain muscle—as long as it's done in partnership with exercise. Yes, I just used the e-word. If you're familiar with *You Are Your Own Gym* or *Body by You,* you won't faint at the mention of exercise; chances are you're already into body-weight training. If not, hold on and hear me out.

My argument is simple and scientifically proven: we need to move enough so that the calories we consume are used to fuel activity and build lean tissue, instead of storing those calories as fat for future activity. Exercising does a bunch of amazing things to your body, and you've heard them a million times: it expends calories, builds muscle, burns unused fat stores, and ups your metabolic rate.

But here's something you may not know: a consistent workout program will change your eating habits for the better. Regular exercisers experience fewer food cravings, they eat more vegetables, and they're less likely to binge on fattening food. Why is this? Exercise steadies blood sugar levels so that you avoid mood swings and cravings. It also elicits the release of endorphins, or natural chemicals, that send feel-good messages to your brain. This is the very same natural "high" you experience after eating certain foods, like dark chocolate. So for a few hours after exercising, that endorphin rush can fill in for food-induced endorphins. Eating right and exercising regularly are as inseparable as Ben and Jerry . . . okay, maybe not such a good analogy, but you get the picture!

Because exercise is a necessary component of weight loss and healthy body maintenance, you'll find a Body Fuel workout in this book, a brand-new exercise program that is a good starting point if you're unfamiliar with body-weight training. This workout is designed to boost your metabolism, build strength, and develop overall athletic ability exceptionally well for the first couple of months.

Relax: you don't have to huff and puff to the commands of a drill sergeant to get the workout you need, like I did when I was a young, aspiring Special Operations trainee. The Body Fuel workouts take no longer than ten minutes, and you have to do them only three times a week (more only if you want).

Whenever you first start an effective training program (in essence, a new form of stress), very little stimulus is needed to prompt adaptation and produce results, and that's why just ten minutes is enough for the untrained person. To get ongoing results, however, a diet and exercise program needs to change and adapt as you change and get stronger and more defined.

Thus, after the first couple of months, switch to one of the workout programs in my previous books. *You Are Your Own Gym* is a great program for all-around fitness but offers a higher-level workout when you're ready for it. *Body by You* presents workouts that develop a solid foundation of strength, and therefore fitness, with a very gradual and progressive body-weight strength training program. I developed *Body by You* with the female body in mind, but it's a great resource for both genders.

As I mentioned earlier, none of my workouts require any fancy equipment, daunting machines, or weird contraptions or gadgets to squeeze. You'll use the best workout "machine" ever designed: your body. Using your body's own resistance, you'll develop greater strength, power, muscular and cardiovascular endurance, tone, and definition, than you ever thought possible. My workouts can be done anywhere, anytime, and without costly gym memberships or equipment. For those of you who are already active, perhaps lifting weights, consider this workout a valuable addition that can be done anywhere, anytime. The exercises work for everyone, no matter what your present level of fitness. It may take a few weeks to see positive results on your waistline and other body parts, but you'll immediately feel more alert, energetic, and in charge of your body. Combined with this diet, the body-weight workout in this book will reward you with the body you want.

I believe that to lose weight and keep it off, you must truly change the way you live. Don't be scared that I'm going to ask you to turn your life upside down and give up everything you love. Quite the opposite. I'm going to give you a clear, simple plan to follow, a way to change the way you think about food, and encouragement as you begin this life- and body-changing experience.

Okay . . . movie trailer over. It's time to look at the big picture.

PART 1

MASTER THE SCIENCE OF A FIRM, FAT-FREE BODY

CHAPTER 1

CARBS: SLOW FUELS AND FAST FUELS

When low-carb dieting was all the rage, sneaking a slice of bread might get you sentenced to hard time. I don't know about you, but I'm glad those days are pretty much over. There's a time and place for all types of carbohydrates, which is why I don't subscribe to the good-carb, bad-carb approach to eating.

I prefer to look at carbs as "slow" or "fast"—based on the speed at which the body absorbs them. Let me explain this distinction and why it's important.

All carbohydrates must be converted to glucose, a type of sugar, before they are absorbed into the bloodstream. Carbs are absorbed at either a fast rate or a slow rate. That rate of absorption produces a proportionately strong release of the hormone insulin, which regulates the amount of sugar in the blood. When we eat carbs that absorb *quickly* (fast carbs), such as candy, soda, or fruit juice, an insulin surge rapidly depletes blood sugar and converts these carbs to fat. We're also left feeling tired, and we crave more food to restore normal blood sugar levels. There's a positive exception to this scenario, though: eating some fast-fuel carbs during or immediately after intense exercise replenishes depleted muscles and aids in the recovery process.

By contrast, slow carbs such as vegetables are absorbed more slowly and do not produce this fat-gaining insulin reaction. Slow-fuel carbs also tend to be high in fat-burning fiber and packed with many more vitamins and minerals than fast-fuel carbs.

GLYCEMIC INDEX VERSUS GLYCEMIC LOAD

How can you tell which carbs are fast-fuel and which are slow-fuel?

I like to use a tool called the *glycemic load*, or GL. GL is a numerical ranking system for carbs that looks at two issues: the amount of carbohydrates in a standard serving of food, say a banana or a cup of rice, and how fast or slow the carbohydrate in that food is released into the bloodstream.

Now, you might be thinking: "Is the glycemic load the same as the glycemic index?" No—but they are related. Like GL, the *glycemic index*, or GI, indicates how quickly carbs dismantle into sugar in your bloodstream. However, the GI does not consider how much carbohydrate there is in a particular serving—in other words, the amount you actually eat.

Just because a carb is high on the index doesn't always indicate that a typical serving of it will hike up your blood sugar level as quickly as its index number makes it seem, because some foods with fast-absorbing sugars do not contain a lot of total carbs per serving.

Here are two examples: Watermelon ranks high on the GI scale at 72. But it has a low GL of 7.21. That high GI is figured on 5 cups of watermelon, not on the typical serving size of 1 cup. The low GL indicates that 1 cup of watermelon doesn't hold much carbohydrate, and that's because it's mostly water. Thus, a serving of watermelon won't jack up your blood sugar the way its index rank might suggest.

Carrots are another example. Carrots have a high GI of 131, so you'd think they would really hike your blood sugar, right? Wrong. That high GI is based on eating a pound and a half of carrots. That's not a normal serving. I mean, really, who crunches down that many carrots? The GL for a typical serving of carrots

(1 carrot) is only 6.5. Therefore, unless you're going to scarf down a massive amount of carrots in one sitting, an average serving of carrots won't hike up your blood sugar.

So you see, the GL is the best indicator of what a particular food does to your blood sugar. The lower the GL of a food, the better it is for weight control and overall health.

FUEL RATINGS: FROM SLOW TO FAST

You don't have to memorize the GL numbers of foods. I've done this for you by dividing all carbohydrate-containing foods on this diet into one of two glycemic load categories:

Slow-fuel carbs. Low-glycemic-load carbs are "slow fuel." They are digested more slowly and therefore provide a smaller amount of longer-lasting energy. They don't jack up insulin levels abnormally—a response that can trigger fat gain or muscle growth after intense training. Slow-fuel carbs have a GL rating of 1 to 6, and they include all low-calorie, high-fiber vegetables such as greens, salad vegetables, broccoli, cauliflower, green beans, yellow squash, zucchini, and so forth. These can be eaten with reckless abandon at any time.

Fast-fuel carbs. All remaining types of carbs—those with a GL of 7 or higher—are considered fast-fuel carbs. They stimulate a greater insulin release and are digested and absorbed quickly by the body. Examples of high-GL carb foods include grain-based products, potatoes, rice, fruit, fruit juice, sports drinks, and sodas. Fast fuels need to be selected carefully and eaten at the right time. I'll show you how to choose the best ones and when to eat them.

INSULIN 101

All carbs have varying effects on the hormone insulin. I'll be mentioning insulin a lot in this book, so I thought we'd take a little detour here and study up on it.

When it comes to getting in shape, insulin can be your best buddy—or your worst enemy.

Insulin's main job is to drive glucose into your cells (including muscle cells) to be burned for energy. It is also an *anabolic* hormone, meaning that it helps you develop lean muscle. But it has a more devilish side: it can increase the storage of body fat. Truth be told, you need to raise insulin levels to develop muscle, but you also need to tamp it down to burn body fat. This all sounds crazy and baffling, so I want to set the record straight.

After you eat a meal of carbs and/or protein, your pancreas churns out insulin. The hormone then enters your bloodstream and journeys to various bodily tissues, including your muscles. The outer perimeters of muscle cells are dotted with insulin receptors, which act like doorbells. Once insulin "rings" the receptor, the muscle cell opens the "door" to allow glucose and amino acids in. The entry of insulin into muscles also activates biochemical reactions that promote the construction of muscle tissue. Insulin has a protective function: it guards against muscle breakdown.

Okay, if insulin is so key for developing lean muscle, how can it also be disadvantageous? Answer: If you overeat carbs, too much insulin pours into the bloodstream. When this happens, the insulin glut increases enzymes responsible for storing fat. This scenario interferes with the body's ability to burn fat for energy, and it stimulates your appetite.

Because insulin can be both positive and negative, it's important to manage it in order to gain muscle *and* lose body fat. Follow these four guidelines, and you'll keep insulin in check.

1. Pay Attention to Glycemic Load

Carb selection can hinder or help your ability to manage insulin. Fast-fuel carbs trigger a blast in blood sugar, which in turn stimulates the release of insulin. This is something you don't want if you're overweight or obese. With the Body Fuel way, you'll learn how and when to eat slow-fuel and fast-fuel carbs to better regulate your body's insulin reaction. For a list of fast-fuel carbs, refer to page 35.

2. Concentrate on Mostly Lower-GL Carbs for Weight Loss

At most of your meals every day, you want to include slow-fuel carbs. These carbs enter the bloodstream gradually and pass more slowly through the digestive system. All of this keeps insulin levels low. You find a long list of all the allowable slow-fuel carbs on page 33.

Slow-fuel carbs are also low in calories and high in fiber—properties that fight weight gain and promote weight control. You can fill up on slow-fuel carbs because their calorie counts are negligible. You stay full longer and can resist the "urge to splurge" on fattening foods. Plus, the fiber in slow-fuel carbs is a true anti-obesity weapon. The less processed and the more natural the food (like slow-fuel carbs), the fewer calories and fat your body absorbs. The fiber also keeps you feeling full, so you don't overeat.

3. Understand When to Use Fast-Fuel Carbs

There are two key times during the day when fast-fuel carbs can help you. The first is upon waking. During sleep, you've fasted for six to eight hours. This overnight fast depletes glycogen—the carbohydrate stored in your muscles and liver. Unless you break the fast, your body will start breaking down muscle tissue for fuel—a bad scenario if you're trying to develop muscle or burn fat. Eating a fast-fuel carb shortly after you awaken will crank out insulin and rapidly replenish your glycogen levels to halt the possible assault on your muscles. I'll show you how and when to do this for best results.

The second time to take in fast-fuel carbs is about thirty to forty-five minutes after your workout. If you're active and training hard, it's okay—and indeed a good idea—to include fast-fuel carbs in your diet, *especially if you're trying to gain strength and muscle mass.*

Fast-fuel carbs quickly restock glycogen after exercise, for three reasons. First, your blood flow is elevated, so carbs get into your system rapidly. Second, your muscles and liver are more receptive to insulin at this time, so insulin can get to work to restock glycogen in your muscles. Third, other enzymes and hormones active in muscle repair and growth have peaked at this time. If you delay—say, for a couple of hours or longer—these enzymes and hormones fall by nearly two-thirds and keep falling from there, and your body quickly moves from an anabolic state (building muscle) to a catabolic state (cannibalizing muscle for protein and fuel). So don't miss this important window of metabolic opportunity. Good post-workout refueling choices include brown rice, whole-grain bread, pasta, potatoes, or smoothies.

4. Employ a Protein Helper After Your Workout

It's best to pair some protein with a fast-fuel carb after your workout, too. Why protein?

While fast-fuel carbs are your premium post-workout fuel, protein is like the handyman who arrives to fix the damage using amino acids. The amino acids help repair your muscles and assist your body in proper recovery. Including protein in a post-workout snack, meal, or smoothie can initiate these processes more quickly than eating just carbs by themselves.

During the thirty- to forty-five-minute window of opportunity after your workout, protein synthesis proceeds at its most efficient rate. This is due to the micro-trauma (breaking down of muscle tissue) that occurred during your workout. Your muscles are craving protein for repair at this time. You'll optimize your recovery if you provide your muscles with amino acids (the key components of protein) after your training session and with a shuttling system to transport the needed nutrients. Protein, along with some carbs, after a workout also creates a hormonal environment that is conducive (and even necessary) to muscular growth and development. More on how to choose proteins in Chapter 2.

FUELING STRATEGIES

Along with quality sources of protein, eating the Body Fuel way includes a mix of slow-fuel carbs and fast-fuel carbs. You'll learn how to think strategically about when to eat these two types of carbs.

Choosing your carbs doesn't stop there, though. I'm going to show you how to select carbs based on their nutritional value. A potential problem with many fast-fuel carbs like table sugar isn't just their spiked insulin response, it's also that they provide few vitamins, minerals, fiber, or other healthful components.

Ideally, the carbs you eat should be as close to their original form as possible, such as whole pieces of fruit, raw or steamed vegetables, and steel-cut oats. Much of our obesity problem in Western civilization can be attributed to consuming massive amounts of highly processed carbs that are high on the glycemic scale and offer little or no nutritional value.

Also, many people mistakenly believe that they can eat whatever food they want as long as it's low in fat, regardless of its glycemic effect or rating, nutritional value, and calorie content. Have you noticed that there are more "healthy" and "low-fat" packaged foods, from cookies and yogurts to sports bars and sodas, than I can count in a lifetime, but we're certainly not getting thinner by eating them? That's because they're packed with sugars and processed carbs to fill in for the fat. And the lack of dietary fat allows all that extra sugar to absorb even faster, creating a stronger insulin reaction, and thus causing people to gain even more body fat.

As long as you remember a few basics about carbs—strategically choosing the less processed, more natural types with a low glycemic load—you'll be well on your way to managing a diet that will get you lean and fit, and keep you there.

CHAPTER 2

THE OTHER BODY FUELS: PROTEIN AND FAT

Trying to lose body fat while developing muscle is a metabolic challenge. You need to manage calories for fat loss, while still supplying enough carbohydrates to fuel your body for exercise. Plus, you need to figure in two other major nutrients—protein to build muscle and fat to help you absorb vitamins and minerals and keep your cells in working order.

PROTEIN FUEL

Protein drives your muscle development and fat-burning mechanisms, particularly when coupled with regular exercise. Protein foods include beef, poultry, fish, eggs, and beans. After you eat protein, it's broken down into amino acids, the building blocks used to repair and regenerate all cells. One of these amino acids is called leucine, and it seems to be the best of the bunch. Your muscles use it as fuel. It helps you develop and maintain lean muscle mass, enabling your body to burn more calories for a boost in weight loss. Animal-based proteins are very high in leucine.

Protein activates your body's fat-burning mechanisms in another way: by helping to produce a hormone called glucagon. Glucagon is like an instant message to your body, directing it to move dietary fat out of storage and into your bloodstream, where it can be burned for fuel.

Also, if you don't eat enough protein, your metabolism can slow down. Muscle is metabolic tissue that requires calories, so if your body dismantles muscle to fulfill its protein requirements, you're losing a key factor in fat burning.

Protein helps you feel full, too, by boosting levels of a hormone called peptide YY, which is obviously of benefit when you're restricting food to lose weight. When you're thinking about taking down some sweets or you're craving carbs, eat a small bite of protein instead. More than likely, your hunger will disappear.

There are other benefits to eating protein. The energy (calories) from protein is used to develop and repair all the body's tissues, especially the muscles. Proteins regulate your body's water balance. Protein is also key to the manufacture of red blood cells, enzymes, hormones, and antibodies that are essential for the proper functioning of your body.

You're going to eat more protein on my plan than you might be used to. It should be the center of every meal.

How Much Protein?

I advise eating 3 to 6 ounces of protein with every main meal. That amount of protein approximates the size of your fist. So play up protein—and watch your body change for the better.

FAT FUEL

By now, you've probably gathered that a major goal of my plan is to maximize lean body mass and minimize body fat. It might surprise you to learn that the typical low-fat diet will not accomplish this; you actually need to eat a diet slightly *higher in fat.*

The very latest word on this comes from a study published in September 2014 in the *Annals of Internal Medicine*. Researchers assigned a group of 150 men and women to follow a diet for one year that was either low-carb (less than 40 grams of carbs daily) and higher in fat or low in fat.

It turned out that the low-carb/higher-fat dieters lost about eight pounds more on average than those on the low-fat diet. The low-carb/higher fat dieters had significantly greater reductions in body fat, too, than the low-fat dieters, and improvements in lean muscle mass—even though neither group changed their exercise level. In fact, the weight lost by the low-fat dieters was mostly muscle mass. I was encouraged after reading these results, since the Body Fuel plan supplies a bit more fat than most diets.

There are two general types of dietary fat: saturated and unsaturated. Saturated fat comes mainly from animal sources, with the exception of coconut oil, which is saturated. Unsaturated fats are derived mainly from plant sources such as nuts, seeds, avocados, olive oil, flaxseed oil, and fish.

Saturated fat has gotten an ill-deserved bad reputation over the years, taking the rap for everything from obesity to heart disease. Yet as long as you don't eat saturated fat to excess, it isn't as harmful as once thought, not even to the heart. Research even supports the principle that diets higher in saturated fat don't always lead to heart disease. A case in point: a study published in the *American Journal of Clinical Nutrition* in 2010 reviewed and analyzed multiple clinical trials of saturated fat and concluded that the real culprit in obesity and heart disease is the amount of carbohydrate people are eating. The study pointed out the following:

- When people lowered saturated fat in their diets but increased carbs (especially refined carbs), they suffered from elevated triglycerides and LDL cholesterol (the artery-clogging type). Both conditions are risk factors for heart disease.
- Substituting saturated fat for carbs actually raised HDL cholesterol (that's the good cholesterol that keeps your arteries clean).

I'd like to add that eating some saturated fat is vital for active people because it helps maintain concentrations of testosterone circulating in the body. Testosterone helps develop muscle growth and promote strength. Research has shown that men who get less than 30 percent of their calories from fat produce 25 percent less testosterone than those who have more fat in their diets.

Nutritional researchers have also observed that over the past four decades, Americans have slashed the percentage of calories they obtain from dietary fat, but ironically, rates of overweight and obesity have risen dramatically. Why? Because too many people are following low-fat diets, replacing fat with highly processed carbs, which are proving to be the real bad guy: the body absorbs them much faster, and they lead to fat *gain*.

So you see, saturated fat isn't the health devil it is made out to be.

Don't get me wrong: I'm not advocating that you go out and start packing away bacon, butter, and marbled rib-eyes like there's no tomorrow. Too much of any nutrient is bad for you, especially when it's out of proportion to other vital nutrients. Balance is key.

How Much Fat?

On this diet, fat makes up 25 to 35 percent of your total calorie intake. That fat will come from both saturated and unsaturated sources. A small palmful of nuts and seeds, a bit of healthful oil on your salad, and animal sources of protein will naturally provide you with the right balance of fats. If you're a vegetarian or a vegan, using coconut oil in the diet will provide you with some needed saturated fat.

WATER: THE FORGOTTEN FUEL

Water is to your body what oil is to your car. You need it to run practically every bodily process, including joint movement, muscle contraction, digestion, waste excretion, circulation, and even breathing.

Too often water is an afterthought, and yet no nutrient is more vital or necessary. True, it has no calories or vitamins, and we're seldom aware of its healthful minerals. But nutrition experts rank it ahead of protein, carbohydrates, fat, vitamins, and minerals in terms of importance. Maintaining proper hydration is an essential part of healthy living. Every day, we lose 2 to 3 quarts of water through urination, sweating, and breathing. We have to replace that water.

Want some proof? Consider these stats. A man's body is approximately 60 percent water, and a woman's is about 50 percent. You can survive weeks without food, but only six days without water. When the water in your body is reduced by just 1 percent, you get thirsty. At 5 percent, muscle strength and endurance deteriorate, and you get hot and tired. When the loss reaches 10 percent, expect to feel delirious with blurry vision. At 20 percent, get someone to call the undertaker. You're dead.

Above and beyond staying not dead, there are specific fitness and weight loss benefits to staying hydrated: pumping up the volume of fluid in your body may lead to an increase in fat breakdown (lipolysis) as well as muscle growth. Yes, folks, drinking water can help you lose fat and build muscle, especially if you perform resistance exercise. Sound too good to be true?

A study conducted at California State University in Fullerton found that dehydration, if coupled with resistance exercise, can be detrimental, compromising the action of certain hormones involved in fat burning and muscle growth. Researchers recruited volunteers to complete three identical workouts under three different conditions: normally hydrated, moderately dehydrated, and more severely dehydrated. They then drew volunteers' blood and tested it for testosterone, cortisol, growth hormone, IGF-1, insulin, glucose, and others. Being inadequately hydrated was found to upset testosterone levels in the following way: it elevated cortisol, and excess cortisol prevents testosterone from entering cells—a situation that drives down metabolism. Cortisol also adversely affected the metabolism of carbs and fat, and that can potentially lead to fat gain.

Water is an influential factor in stimulating thermogenesis—a process that, by creating heat in the body, causes you to burn more calories. How many more calories?

If we go by the results of one key study, the answer is about 100. In the particular study, researchers snagged fourteen healthy, normal-weight volunteers (seven men and seven women) and instructed them to drink 500 milliliters of water. That's 17 ounces, a little over two 8-ounce glasses. Just those two glasses increased the volunteers' metabolic rate by 30 percent within a forty-minute period. The researchers estimated that this increase was the equivalent of burning about 25 extra calories. Well, if you drink eight glasses of water a day, you're burning 100 calories, effortlessly and automatically. Water is a true fat burner!

Drinking enough water clearly plays a serious role in fat burning and muscle building. Staying well hydrated also helps your liver efficiently eliminate toxins, and it helps transport nutrients into cells. Water maintains the correct balance of vitamins, minerals, and electrolytes in your system, too. Electrolytes such as sodium, potassium, and chloride help ensure that your muscles and joints can move through their full range of motion, and are resistant to muscle spasms and cramping. They also regulate the pattern of your heartbeat. Other jobs of water are to maintain the proper density of your blood, regulate blood pressure, and move fats so that they don't get deposited as plaque in your blood vessels. Water is a virtual miracle worker in the body.

Dehydration, on the other hand, can lead to sugar cravings, fatigue, and a bad mood marked by edginess and foggy thinking. The first troubleshooting step for just about any malady should be to check your water intake. Everything from headaches, skin problems, and junk food cravings to sore muscles and irritability can be caused by being dehydrated.

How Much Water?

Keeping yourself properly hydrated should be a top priority when you're trying to get in great shape. Aim to drink *at least* 8 cups of pure water a day—even more if you're exercising regularly.

A few years ago, the American College of Sports Medicine (ACSM) published its "Position Stand on Exercise and Fluid Replacement" in its journal *Medicine and Science in Sports and Exercise*. The position paper provided a couple of clear guidelines about when to drink water if you're active:

- Two hours before you exercise: drink about 17 ounces (500 ml) of fluid to hydrate the body and allow excretion of excess fluid.
- During exercise: start drinking early and continue at regular

intervals to try to replace fluid lost through sweating. Weigh yourself before you train and right afterward to determine if you've replaced enough liquid. If you generally lose 3 to 4 pounds during your workout, you need to drink 6 to 8 cups of fluid as you exercise to offset that fluid loss.

To keep it as simple as possible, I suggest that you carry a water bottle with you at all times and keep it filled. Drink a cup of water with every meal or snack, too. Have a glass of water as soon as you get up in the morning, too. I keep a glass of water next to my bed at night and have myself a drink whenever I wake up in the middle of the night. I down the remainder first thing in the morning. These habits will help you automatically get enough water. Never let thirst be your guide, either. By the time you're actually thirsty, you're already dehydrated.

If you're wondering whether you're well hydrated or not, check your pee. If it's consistently colorless or very light, you're drinking enough water.

It is impossible to overemphasize the importance of proper nutrition. A good understanding of these dietary fundamentals, from the glycemic load to the nutrients in foods, is absolutely necessary to reach and sustain your fitness goals. Build an awareness of what you put in your body, and apply these basic principles. Then, by learning and following the Body Fuel way, eventually you'll hardly have to think about it anymore. So far, I've shown you which carbohydrates, proteins, and fats are best. Next, I'm going to show you how to manage these nutrients in an important process called "calorie cycling," the secret weapon underlying this diet.

CHAPTER 3

CALORIE CYCLING

With the exception of water, all the fuels I've just talked about provide calories. Calories are a measurement of how much energy is released when your body breaks down food. Weight gain, weight loss, and weight maintenance are, to a large degree but not exclusively, a matter of calories in versus calories out. Somewhat oversimplified: excess calories are stored as fat, whereas a calorie deficit causes stored fat to be burned as energy.

Most diets are based on restricting calories. The theory goes that if you cut, say, 500 calories a day, you should lose a pound a week, since 1 pound of body weight is equivalent to 3,500 calories (500 calories × 7 days = 3,500 calories).

Calorie restriction does work, but it has limitations, especially if the calorie (fuel) choices are low quality or poorly planned. Constant calorie restriction is nearly impossible to maintain over the long term, because you continuously feel unsatisfied. That's when boredom and deprivation enter the picture, setting you up for failure.

Also, weight loss is often only modest, rather than dramatic, on these diets.

Some research has found that after months and months of dieting, weight loss often slows to a frustrating pace. This is partly due to the fact that your choices in fuels affect how your body metabolizes those calories. Without the right split of macronutrients (carbs, proteins, and fats) and enough of the nutrient-dense slow-fuel carbs, your body is far more likely to use the consumed energy for building fat, rather than building muscle, which causes a metabolic downward spiral, since muscle requires calories even while at rest.

Perhaps the biggest problem with constant calorie restriction is that it slows your resting metabolic rate (RMR). RMR refers to the number of calories your body burns in everyday functions: breathing, the pumping of your heart, fat burning, filtering waste via your kidneys, and so forth. Your RMR accounts for anywhere from 60 percent to 75 percent of the total calories you expend daily—it is the engine of life. The remaining calories are burned through activity.

Here's where overly restrictive diets go wrong. Your body eventually adapts to an ongoing, consistent calorie deficit by turning down the furnace and slowing your metabolic rate. Thus, the more pounds you drop, the fewer calories you need. Why? For one, there is less of you to fuel. Also, the body increases its metabolic efficiency to balance energy input and output. The body is extremely resourceful. During times of starvation—or calorie restriction, which it interprets the same way—it adapts by slowing down the RMR, increasing efficiency. It tries to save every calorie consumed by storing some as fat. It is far less likely to create metabolically expensive tissue like muscle, especially when the demand for physical strength isn't high. A very large part of survival is balancing energy input and output. Your body will adapt to an ongoing calorie deficit by increasing efficiency (do more with less), and that means fat will be favored over muscle, especially if you aren't doing strength training. Most diets that restrict calories neglect this principle, and this is why people on those diets almost always gain their weight back (and sometimes more).

Because some people have a lower RMR (greater efficiency), they have more of a tendency to gain weight than others—great for periods of starvation but not so good in an age of abundance. Conversely, people with higher RMRs (lower efficiency) burn more calories, especially at rest. Ideally, in today's affluent society, you want a high RMR that uses energy freely to lose fat and keep it off. That is what this diet is all about—showing you how to fuel your body to build muscle, be satisfied, stay healthy, and keep the furnace burning on high!

A NEW AND IMPROVED WAY TO BURN FAT AND BUILD MUSCLE

There are a couple of different variables that can affect your RMR, namely, exercise and nutrition. You can manipulate these factors to power up your RMR.

The first and foremost is calorie cycling. Unlike the typical calorie restrictive diet, in which you stick to a static, low-calorie plan, calorie cycling periodically changes your caloric intake up or down. Your calories never stay constant for more than a few weeks on this plan. For example, you'll follow a plan of higher-calorie eating for approximately three weeks (Block 3), followed by two weeks of lower-calorie dieting (Block 2), followed by one week of more intense calorie cutting (Block 1).

When your body receives a differing amount of calories—say, higher calories for a couple of weeks, followed by lower calories for the next couple of weeks—this allows your RMR to remain high, and consequently burn off more calories. In other words, calorie cycling jerks your metabolism around so that it never gets sluggish, but keeps burning fat. This concept is similar to what happens when you change your workout volume and intensity from time to time in order to keep your body adapting to new stimulus. Periodic changes in your caloric intake (volume) and strictness of your fuel choices (intensity) do the same thing.

During the periods of higher caloric volume, you'll have more freedom in your fuel choices (lower dieting intensity). As your caloric volume decreases throughout the three blocks, your choices in fuels diminish somewhat. Just as with my exercise programs, volume and intensity are inversely proportionate and constantly changing.

One big advantage of this is that fixed periods of higher-calorie intake (like in that first, longest block of three weeks and the middle, moderate block of two weeks) is that during these periods you will be able to train harder and recover faster. It's really not possible to make optimal progress with your training while on a constant calorie deficit. You *need* those extra calories from fast fuels in Block 3 and Block 2 if you want to perform at your best and add as much lean, RMR-boosting muscle tissue as possible.

Just as a good training program systematically fluctuates how much and hard you train, your diet should also systematically change the type and quantity of your calories. Calorie cycling leads to more muscle and less fat than if you were to follow the same diet for four weeks straight or longer.

Calorie cycling also prevents diet plateauing, in which you seem to stop losing weight, or you find that your clothes aren't getting looser anymore. You're stuck. Every serious athlete, exerciser, or dieter has been there and done that. With calorie cycling, there's less likelihood of plateauing until you have reached your target weight, because there's more change, and that equals more adaptation.

The second way to increase your RMR is through resistance training, including body-weight exercises. My workouts build lean muscle, and muscle accounts for 80 percent of your RMR. Conversely, body fat is sluggish, inactive, and programmed to use a minimal amount of calories; its role is to insulate you and to act as a storeroom for your future energy supply. Muscle is active, fat-burning tissue. The more you have, the higher your RMR. The Body Fuel workout, beginning on page 193, will get you there.

THE SCIENCE OF CALORIE CYCLING

I know from my own experience and those of my clients that calorie cycling *works.* Need more proof? In 2014, medical researchers in Iran put people on a typical calorie-restricted diet or a calorie-cycling diet. The subjects on the calorie-cycling diet changed their intake from high to low calories to decrease weight, and then changed it from low to high calories to keep their RMR at higher levels.

The outcome of this experiment was quite decisive. Those on the calorie-cycling plan suffered no reduction in RMR, while the calorie-restricting dieters had a significant drop in their RMR. The calorie-cycling group lost more weight and body fat than dieters in the other group, too. Plus, with calorie cycling, dieters reported feeling more satisfied and less hungry than the other calorie-restricted dieters did. Calorie cycling clearly maximizes your metabolism and your results.

CALORIE CYCLING AND YOUR HORMONES

Calorie cycling stimulates your metabolic hormones, too. I'm referring to any hormone that influences fat storage and fat burning, including insulin, growth hormone, testosterone, IGF-1 (a type of growth hormone that is similar to insulin), and thyroid hormones.

Without getting into too much biochemistry, we know from research that:

- When you first lower your caloric and carb intake, your pancreas produces glucagon, the hormone that unlocks fat stores when food is limited. Soon great things begin to happen: unsightly body fat is burned, and you get leaner. This goes on until the body finds a balance between energy input and output by shedding weight and slowing the RMR.
- As I've explained above, most of the calories you'll be shifting come from the carbohydrate camp. And that's what helps you get leaner. When you ease back on carbs, your muscles surrender stored carbohydrates (muscle glycogen) as energy. Generally, when glycogen levels dip, your body cranks up its ability to burn body fat as energy.
- When you increase calories for at least two to three weeks, you trigger rises in testosterone and IGF-1. Testosterone is a male hormone that stimulates muscle growth, but women have a little of it, too. IGF-1 stimulates protein synthesis and prevents muscle loss. So even though you're eating more calories in Block 3, your body has moved into a fat-burning, muscle-building mode when you practice calorie cycling. And this is especially true while using a good strength-training program, like the one in *You Are Your Own Gym* and *Body by You* or the Body Fuel workouts I'm giving you here.

- When you employ calorie cycling, your thyroid function reaps some benefits, too. The butterfly-shaped thyroid gland, which sits in the throat on either side of your windpipe, manufactures and stores hormones that control your metabolism. Thyroid levels can fluctuate with the quantity and quality of your nutrition. For example, dieters on constant calorie-restricted diets often undergo a dip in thyroid levels, while those who fuel themselves adequately experience an increase in thyroid levels. Slightly elevated thyroid levels not only help stimulate fat burning but also increase the development of muscle.

Hoo-ya!

RMR How-To

There are other strategies you can employ to boost your RMR:

- Eat several meals a day. Meal frequency affects your RMR in two major ways. First, every time you eat a meal or a snack, your metabolism goes up—which means that your body is turning that food into fuel. Second, eating multiple meals suppresses cortisol (a hormone that can increase fat around the belly). When cortisol is suppressed, testosterone increases, and your body is able to better preserve its lean muscle.

  Another way of saying the same thing: don't skip meals. If your body gets used to not eating for long stretches, it will adapt by conserving energy and reducing the number of calories it burns. It's a bad idea to regularly "save yourself" for a big dinner by eating nothing during the day. Your RMR will go into starvation mode and your body will burn up fewer of the calories you gorge that evening.

  The bottom line? Five meals—three main meals and two snacks—spaced throughout the day are easier to absorb, will prevent cravings, and will accelerate your RMR in order to help you get leaner. That's what you'll be getting during every block of this plan.

- Don't neglect breakfast. As you sleep, your body uses less energy so it can focus on repairing damage. By the time you wake, your body is in full-on conservation mode and burning calories very slowly. If you don't give it food within an hour of waking, it continues to burn fat slower for the rest of the day. Crank up your fat burning for the day by eating any of my recommended breakfasts.
- Balance your meals. Boost your RMR by eating the right things in the right combinations. As soon as you eat anything, your metabolic rate rises as your body works to digest the food. But to maximize the burn, you need to eat the healthiest carbs, proteins, and fats together. The aim is to extend the energy boost provided by carbs by combining them with proteins and/or fats each time you eat them. Proteins and fats slow the rate at which carbs are digested, which means your RMR stays higher for longer. My meal plans will show you how to do this.
- Veg out. Eat unlimited quantities of slow-fuel vegetables to hike your RMR for minimal calories. These foods shine because they're fiber-rich and encourage the body to use more fat as fuel, issuing a more urgent boost-my-metabolism message. On my plan, you'll have at least three servings of slow-fuel vegetables a day.

Now that you have an understanding of how calorie cycling works, I bet you're wondering whether you'll have to laboriously add and subtract calories on my plan, or look up calorie counts of foods. No. I've done all that work for you. I'm counting the calories. I'm doing the math. Follow the Body Fuel way and you automatically shift your calories for weight loss and muscle building. But it's also very simple to do yourself—eat a portion of protein with each meal, eat as many slow-fuel vegetables as you want, and control the fast-fuel carbs.

Calorie cycling is a potent diet strategy. You can use it to achieve the most elusive aspects of getting in shape: the burning of fat and the simultaneous development of muscle. If you want to get super-fit and firm without getting fat, it's time to give this strategy a whirl. What follows is the nuts and bolts of how to do so!

PART 2

REAL FUEL

CHAPTER 4

WHAT TO EAT: THE MAGNIFICENT 7

Meats. Fish. Eggs. Vegetables. Fruits. Grains. Nuts and seeds.

Meet the seven food groups that form the core of the Body Fuel plan.

For millions of years, early humans lived on these fuels. The women gathered nuts, seeds, fruits, and vegetables for food, while men hunted for meat. Together, these food sources provided the vital nutrients that helped humans thrive. Climate, geography, and luck mainly determined how available these sources were during any given season, but regardless of how much of each food our ancestors ate, these were the only foods available to them, so naturally our bodies have adapted to their consumption.

These foods produce optimum health and really formed the original natural diet. Scientists have found evidence in the fossil records not only that our cave-dwelling ancestors were trim, lean, muscular, and healthy, but also that they did not generally suffer from many of the diseases that plague us today. As long as they weren't gored by wild beasts or killed in war, many lived quite robustly well up into their seventies and eighties. And recently there's been a trend of

Paleolithic-era-inspired diets, often referred to as "paleo," which aim to exclude all things that could not have been hunted or gathered by humans 10,000 to 2.6 million years ago.

Processed foods such as pasta, bread, and dairy didn't come on the scene until about ten to twelve thousand years ago, when we domesticated plants and animals. That's a tiny segment of time compared to the hundreds of thousands of years spent hunting and gathering our food. Other fillers, such as rice and potatoes, were also not available in large amounts until we started planting edible vegetation and raising livestock. This was all good news, and our societies flourished on these new food sources. The problem now is that over the last sixty years, technology has allowed food companies to process many foods even more, taking them farther and farther from their original form, until very little nutritional value remains beyond empty, fattening calories. Overindulgence in these modern foods has hurt human health, plaguing us with diseases unknown to our ancestors, such as obesity, cancer, heart disease, diabetes, Alzheimer's, and various lifestyle maladies.

The relatively long lives many people enjoy today can be attributed largely to medical advancements rather than to good nutrition or healthful living. We're keeping people alive with medicine—statins, blood thinners, surgery, stents, and other medical inventions—who otherwise would have died a long time ago.

In my work with clients, athletes, and military trainees over the years, I've found that the most direct route to an ideal physique (less body fat and more muscle mass) is to rely on foods that are as close to their original form as possible and to reduce our intake of highly processed foods. Because I'm a realist, I'm not saying give them up altogether; I'm just saying think of these new, more processed foods as little more than fillers in the diet that should ideally only be used to improve recovery from intense training.

The foundation of this diet is made up of food that is as close as possible to its original form when it was still alive, whether plant or animal. Take a tour of these foods and learn how they work metabolically in your favor.

THE PROTEIN FUELS

Meats

This fuel category includes lean meats and poultry. All are superb sources of protein. Remember, protein protects muscle and enhances metabolic hormones. It is also a fat burner and a natural appetite suppressant. The amount of protein you'll eat on my plan is excellent for building, repairing, and preserving lean muscle.

YOUR MEAT CHOICES

Beef:

Arm chuck pot roast	Lean ground beef	Sirloin
Bison	New York strip	Tenderloin
Bottom round	Prime rib	Top loin
Eye round	Rib-eye	

Lamb:

Breast	Leg	Roast
Chops, all types		

Pork:

Canadian bacon	Cutlet	Loin roast
Chop	Ham	Tenderloin

Veal:

Breast	Shoulder arm roast	Sirloin steak
Chops	Shoulder arm steak	
Roast, all types	Shoulder blade steak	

Venison:

All cuts

Poultry:

Chicken breast
Dark meat chicken, including thighs and legs
Cornish hen
Ground chicken
Quail
Turkey breast
Dark meat turkey
Turkey sausage or turkey bacon

Hoo-ya!

Grass-Fed Versus Grain-Fed

One vital and often overlooked factor of our well-being is the health of the animals (and plants) we consume. It's important to consider the methods used to grow or raise our food and also the process used to get that food into our hands, because ultimately the health of the livestock we eat affects our health. For this reason, I'm conscious and cautious about whether the meat I eat is grass-fed rather than grain-fed. With the exception of mother's milk before weaning, this means that the cattle were raised entirely eating grass from pastures, as opposed to being fed with grain. Why is grass-fed better? Meat from grass-fed livestock:

- Has fewer calories
- Is packed with more vitamin E, beta-carotene, and vitamin C
- Is richer in omega-3 fatty acids
- Contains a higher concentration of conjugated linoleic acid, or CLA—a "good" fat that may strengthen immunity, normalize blood sugar, and help fat burning in the body
- Is unlikely to contain any additives, including chemicals, pesticides, growth hormones, or genetically modified feed

It's also smart to shop for meat that is labeled "organic." Animals raised organically have not been given hormones or antibiotics to promote growth. Although they may have eaten only organic feed, they may not be grass-fed, however. When you're shopping for healthful meat, the best choice is to look for meat labeled both certified organic and grass-fed.

Fish and Shellfish

Fish is an excellent source of protein, too, and it's also loaded with omega-3 fatty acids. These amazing fats have the power to affect fat metabolism, diverting it away from storage and burning it for energy. If your belly runneth over, eat fish, particularly salmon and tuna. Both are high in omega-3 fats, known to help reduce abdominal fat. There's more: a 2013 study in the medical journal *Diabetes* revealed that fish oil can actually shrink the size of fat cells—a phenomenon that contributes to a trimmer body.

YOUR FISH AND SHELLFISH CHOICES

Bass
Catfish
Clams
Cod
Flounder
Grouper
Haddock
Mahi-mahi
Monkfish
Mussels
Orange roughy
Oysters
Perch
Redfish
Red snapper
Salmon
Sardines, canned without oil
Scallops
Shark
Shrimp
Tilapia
Trout
Tuna, fresh or canned without oil
Whitefish

Hoo-ya!

Should You Worry About Mercury?

Are there dangerous mercury levels in fish, you ask? I know people who are so afraid of eating fish that they wear hazmat suits in seafood restaurants. It turns out that a lot of this fear might be unfounded. A 2013 study by the University of Bristol suggests that fish accounts for only 7 percent of mercury levels in our bodies, with all food and drink totaling less than 17 percent. Surprisingly, the study also found that herbal teas and alcohol were linked to the highest mercury blood levels, after white and oily fish. I love fish, and I know its omega-3 fats are food for my heart and my physique, so I was pleasantly surprised to learn that it accounts for such a minute amount of blood mercury levels.

Sometimes I think we obsess too much on supposedly dangerous stuff in our foods, but not the other stuff that studies show can make us really sick, such as aspartame, high-fructose corn syrup, and trans fats. Those are the real killers. Yet we bring them into our homes by the carload.

I'm not a knee-jerk fitness person, and I don't give knee-jerk advice. Eating fish is all about moderation. It's fine to go with seafood with lower mercury levels, like salmon, shrimp, and tilapia. Other fish such as swordfish and white tuna have higher levels of mercury. My recommendation: enjoy a grilled shark steak or a tuna sandwich a couple of times a month, not daily.

Eggs

Eggs have been nicknamed the "perfect food." They are a high-quality source of protein and contain a number of vitamins and minerals. Eggs also have an extremely high biological value, which means that the body absorbs and retains egg protein completely and efficiently. Plus, they have been shown to help control appetite.

YOUR EGG CHOICES

Eggs, all varieties
Egg whites
Egg substitute

THE CARBOHYDRATE FUELS

Slow-Fuel Vegetables

This diet is full of natural vitamins, minerals, and fiber (that all-time great fat burner) found in a wide variety of slow-fuel vegetables. These foods have the lowest glycemic load and the lowest caloric count of other foods. Certain slow-fuel vegetables positively affect your hormones for better fat burning, too. These are cruciferous vegetables like broccoli, cauliflower, Brussels sprouts, cabbage, and kale, among others. All of these veggies have phytochemicals that can rein in fat-promoting estrogens and lessen their negative impact on testosterone levels.

For decades, experts, including our parents and grandparents, have been saying that vegetables are good for us. They're right: veggies protect us from all sorts of life-shortening diseases. So if the thought of dying young scares you, eat your slow-fuel veggies. On this plan, you can eat liberal amounts of these foods.

YOUR SLOW-FUEL VEGETABLE CHOICES

Arugula
Asparagus
Beet greens
Bok choy
Broccoli
Broccoli rabe
Brussels sprouts
Cabbage, all types
Celery
Collard greens
Cucumber
Dandelion greens
Eggplant
Endive
Garlic
Green beans
Kale
Lettuce, all types
Mushrooms, all types
Mustard greens
Okra
Onions
Parsley
Pea pods
Peppers, all types
Scallions
Spinach
Sprouts (alfalfa, broccoli, mung, and so forth)
Summer squash
Swiss chard
Tomatoes
Turnip greens
Water chestnuts
Watercress
Yellow beans
Zucchini

Hoo-ya!

Get Jazzed About Juicing

Sometimes people will tell me that they don't like vegetables. So I suggest that they try juicing. Juicing is an easy way to get a lot of different types of vegetables into your body right away. In doing so, you get an instant surge of vitamins and minerals. Fresh juices contain digestive enzymes that work to scrub away toxins in your digestive tract, revitalizing your entire system. They're also loaded with phytochemicals, natural substances in plants that promote good health and defend the body against diseases.

Another reason I promote juicing on this plan is that it helps fight food cravings. If you've tried to lose weight in the past but felt hungry for sweets and other foods all the time, it could be because you lacked some essential vitamins and minerals. Juicing helps replenishes those elements and satisfy a sweet tooth. The net effect is that you may eat less of the wrong foods, save calories, and thus lose weight.

A downside is that juicing removes fiber content, unless you're using only a blender to pulverize the veggies. So it's always wise to put some of that removed fiber back into your juice. Add some plant-based protein powder and oils to your juice, too; those help control blood sugar spikes.

Some tips to improve your juicing experience:

- Juice mainly vegetables, including leafy greens (which boast some of the highest concentrations of vitamins and phytochemicals). For greens, try cabbage, kale, or spinach, and toss in a little parsley (helps purify the blood) or cilantro (helps detoxify heavy metals).
- Go easy on fruit juice. It can be too concentrated with sugar and may affect your insulin response negatively. Instead, use fruit only as a flavoring for your juices, and allow the vegetables to take center stage. A good sweetening fruit is green apple. Carrots and beets are good sweeteners, but use them judiciously.
- Drink it right away. Juiced produce rapidly loses its nutritional power and becomes prone to spoilage. So plan to drink your juice immediately after making it. If you

need to wait for a few hours, pour it into a container, tightly affix the lid, and keep it refrigerated.

As for a juicer, base your selection on its mechanism of action, as well as your budget. There are three kinds of juicers: centrifugal, masticating, and triturating. Centrifugal are the least expensive—and the least effective. They produce some heat and remove the most fiber from produce. Masticating machines are the midprice option, and they're believed to preserve a little more of the fiber. Triturating juicers are the most expensive—and the most effective. They press the produce to extract the maximum amount of juice.

For a great juice, try my Fuelin' Veggie Juice on page 158.

Fast-Fuel Vegetables

The choices below are categorized as fast-fuel vegetables because their glycemic load and calorie count per serving are higher than those of the veggies listed earlier. Fast-fuel carbs are also slightly higher in starch content, which is why they are often referred to as "starchy vegetables."

YOUR FAST-FUEL VEGETABLE CHOICES

Beans and legumes:

Black beans
Broad beans
Chickpeas (garbanzos)
Cranberry beans
Great northern beans
Kidney beans
Lentils
Lima beans
Navy beans
Pink beans
Pinto beans
White beans

Beets
Carrots
Corn
Parsnips
Peas
Sweet potatoes
Turnips
Winter squash

Fast-Fuel Fruits

I classify all fruits as fast fuels, because they contain simple sugars and have a higher glycemic load than slow fuels. Fruits tend to be high in fiber, which slows their digestion for better hunger management and weight control than other sources of sweet, simple sugars. Plus, these foods are loaded with antioxidants and other natural substances that keep your body in peak health.

Fruit can help satisfy a sweet tooth, if you have one, and this can go a long way when you're trying to lose body fat. Any and all fruits are fine; I don't think you need to rule any one type out entirely, like some diets do. Most of my clients like some fruit with their breakfast, but it can be eaten at any meal where fast fuels are indicated. It's good right before or during workouts for energy, too, and afterward, to replenish glycogen. Unlike slow-fuel vegetables, though, fruit is not a free food. Fruit still falls under the umbrella of carbs that must be controlled.

The other thing I advise people about regarding fruit is the risk associated with pesticides and hormones. If you're eating fruit that doesn't have a thick peel, such as an apple or berries, buy organic and wash them well. Fruits that do have thick peels are pretty well protected by the peels themselves, so I don't think you need to spend the extra money on, for example, organic bananas or oranges.

YOUR FRUIT CHOICES

Apples
Apricot
Bananas

Berries:

Blackberries
Blueberries
Cranberries
Raspberries
Strawberries

Cherries
Dried fruit
Grapefruit
Grapes
Guava
Mango
Melon, all varieties
Nectarines
Oranges

Papayas
Peaches
Pears
Pineapple
Plums
Tangelos
Tangerines
Watermelon

Fast-Fuel Grains

Many fans of the paleo fad claim that our ancestors did not eat grains. But they mostly certainly did, at least some of the time, depending on where they lived and what time period you're talking about. In fact, they were constantly gathering grain-based foods like wild wheat. Though the pursuit of meat was pretty constant, for many the kill was infrequent. They didn't sit down to mammoth chops at every meal or even every dinner.

Too often we generalize and wind up labeling an entire category of food as being "bad." Grain products are definitely one of those categories that have gotten a bad rap. They are not all the same, and it's important that you distinguish between good grains and lesser grains.

For example, if a piece of bread can be turned into a ball of dough by squeezing it in your hand, it should probably be avoided unless you're looking for a quick post-workout sugar and insulin boost to replenish lost glycogen stores. Here's why: to make such a fine, white-grain product, the bran (hard outer shell) and the germ (reproductive part) of whole grains are removed during a mechanical grinding process in which the vitamins and fiber are taken out, leaving only the fast-absorbed sugars. Bleach and other chemicals are then added to further soften and whiten the grain.

These highly refined and processed grains are what make up the bulk of grain products found packaged in grocery stores, and they are largely responsible for our weight and health problems. But this does not make all grain products bad, especially if you're fairly active and exercise regularly! You'll want to include the healthier, far less processed grain choices in your diet to fuel hard workouts and to help you recover properly, so you can get the most benefit possible from every squat, lunge, press, and pull. Don't go completely grain dead on me: making smart grain selections is easy.

On this diet, grains are classified as fast fuels. Of all foods, they're highest in carbohydrate, with the highest potential to raise insulin and blood sugar. You'll eat them in limited quantities (even whole-grain bread); it is not wise to omit them altogether. We need a variety of whole grains, as well as legumes, fruits, and vegetables, in order to get the gamut of dietary fibers required for the health of the heart and digestive system, as well as for the regulation of insulin and glucose. And if you're a vegan or a vegetarian, the different types of fibers and amino acids in grain and legumes make them a perfect nutritional match.

If you're cutting out gluten, choose gluten-free grains; they're marked with an asterisk in the list below. Gluten-free goes along with my recommendation to eat as many of our ancestors did. It wasn't until about ten thousand years ago, when people began domesticating crops, that the gluten in our diets increased dramatically, and in some parts of the world, its consumption is still relatively low. As a result, a lot of people don't have the needed digestive enzymes required to break it down.

YOUR FAST-FUEL GRAIN CHOICES

An asterisk (*) indicates gluten-free grains.

*Amaranth
*Brown rice
*Buckwheat
Couscous
Instant or quick-cooking oatmeal
*Millet
Pastas
Pearled barley
*Quinoa
Ready-to-eat cereals
Sprouted bread
Steel-cut oats
100 percent whole-grain bread
*White rice
*Wild rice

Post-Workout Fast Fuels

Some of you will be able to metabolically handle foods that are a bit higher in sugar and starch. You are in this group if:

- You work out very intensely on a regular basis (three to seven times weekly)
- You have a job that could be described as highly active, such as in construction

- You are a "hard gainer," meaning that you have a hard time gaining weight, especially muscle mass

If you are in any one of these groups, you'll benefit by consuming carbs with a higher sugar content. These fast-fuel carbs will spike blood glucose faster, optimizing muscle glycogen repletion and a hormonal environment necessary for muscle building. Examples of fast-fuel carbs include 8 ounces of a sports drink, an energy bar, a plain baked potato, a bagel, or a peanut butter and jelly sandwich on white bread.

THE FAT FUELS

Nuts, Seeds, and Other Fats

You'll be getting some saturated fats from meats and omega-3 fats from fish, but you'll also obtain fats from nuts and seeds. High in unsaturated fats, nuts and seeds are packed with fiber, protein, and beneficial antioxidants. They're also brimming with glutamine, an amino acid that helps spare lean muscle. Nuts and seeds are good appetite regulators, too. (Just don't stuff yourself with them, because they are very high in calories.) The Body Fuel plan includes not only raw nuts and seeds but also nut butters. These foods are good sources of protein as well.

I also recommend that you eat 1 tablespoon daily of either olive oil, flaxseed oil, or coconut oil (a plant source of saturated fat). These are advantageous because instead of being easily packed as body fat, they enhance muscle growth and fat burning.

YOUR NUT AND SEED CHOICES*

Almonds	Nut butters, any type	Pumpkin seeds
Brazil nuts	Peanuts	Sesame seeds
Cashews	Pecans	Sunflower seeds
Macadamia nuts	Pistachio nuts	Walnuts

*The serving size for nuts and seeds is roughly a handful; for nut butters, 1 tablespoon.

BONUS FUELS

I'm a fan of protein shakes, and you can enjoy them on this diet as an in-between meal snack. To me, whipping up a protein shake is how cooking should be: quick and easy with very little cleanup. Toss a bunch of healthful stuff in the blender, punch a button, and seconds later you're in business. Also, studies have consistently proven that when protein shakes are taken before and after workouts, muscle growth and the hormones that contribute to muscle-growth potential are enhanced.

The protein shakes on my plan are made with two bases: nondairy milks (almond, coconut, rice, or soy milks) and a plant-based protein powder. These powders are typically formulated with brown rice, pea, hemp, or quinoa proteins. (If you'd rather not go with plant-based protein powders, I suggest you try a whey protein powder. Whey is an ingredient with some terrific fat-burning and muscle-building perks.)

To these bases, you can add fresh fruit or green leafy vegetables such as spinach or kale; plus your daily allotment of flaxseed, olive, or coconut oil.

There are several guidelines to bear in mind when choosing a plant-based protein powder. First, look at the label. The very first ingredient should be the vegetable protein source. Second, read the label again to make sure that it's free of genetically modified ingredients (GMOs), sugar, fructose, and any artificial flavor. Third, I don't recommend that you choose a protein powder made with soy. Soy can mess with your hormonal balance over time and isn't good for weight control. Finally, an organic blend is a healthful choice when you're looking at different brands.

In the recipe section starting on page 120, I've got some delicious smoothie and shake recipes for you, all using plant-based protein powders, and I'll show you how to incorporate them into your meal planning.

BODY FUEL CONDIMENTS

Make sure your pantry and fridge hold a collection of diet-friendly condiments:

- All-fruit jams
- Barbecue sauce (if it's low in sugar)
- Herbs and spices
- Honey (in very small amounts)
- Horseradish
- Hot sauces
- Ketchup
- Lemon juice
- Lime juice
- Mayonnaise (fat-free or low-fat varieties)
- Mustard, all types
- Nonstick vegetable sprays
- No-sugar-added pasta or marinara sauce
- Relish
- Salad dressings (fat-free or low-fat varieties; homemade is best, in which you mix vinegar and spices with olive oil)
- Salsa
- Soy sauce (reduced-sodium)
- Steak sauce
- Teriyaki sauce
- Vinegars

Hoo-ya!

If You're a Vegan or Vegetarian

With a few easy tweaks to the Body Fuel plan, vegans and vegetarians will have no problem following this style of eating. Of the Magnificent 7, the foods that fit easily into a plant-based diet include vegetables, fruits, grains, nuts, seeds, and eggs if you're a vegetarian who includes them. Good vegetable sources of protein include legumes, soy proteins such as tofu, and nuts, nut butters, and seeds. In Chapter 9, on page 160, I'll provide some sample meals to show you how to substitute vegetable proteins for animal proteins. It's not difficult to get the protein and other nutrients you need on this plan as a vegan or vegetarian.

MARKED FOODS

I mentioned earlier that my diet isn't exclusionary. Although I prefer to focus on all the foods you can have, rather than those to avoid, you will, however, want to become a stranger to some foods. I call these "Marked Foods."

Dairy

Growing up, I had some allergies. My parents attributed them to all the milk I was drinking. So as a kid I drank mostly almond or soy milk and ate it on my cereal. Even today, too much dairy leaves me feeling a little gassy. When I first got out of the Air Force, a few of my buddies suffered slightly from irritable bowel syndrome (IBS). I suggested they cut out dairy foods, along with wheat products. Within two days, their IBS was gone. Also, I find that whenever I'm eating an Asian-based diet, as I did while training at Thai boxing camps in Thailand—rice, protein, and veggies—my digestive system runs like a charm. If you think about it, we are the only species of animal that drinks the milk of another species, and most people around the world haven't been doing it for very long.

What a lot of people don't realize is that milk products, especially low-fat versions, produce high insulin responses, despite being low-glycemic foods. This is because milk and dairy foods contain lactose, a sugar. In a study published in the *American Journal of Clinical Nutrition*, dairy products triggered similar or greater insulin responses than white bread. Remember, too much of an insulin response can create a fat-forming environment in the body. I've observed that when people cut out or ease back on dairy, they often get more lean and muscular.

Artificial Sweeteners

I consider artificial sweeteners a Marked Food, too. They can make you fat—even the occasional diet soda. Fake sweeteners cause many of the same reactions that regular sugar does, because the receptors on your tongue and in your stomach can't discern between real sugar and fake sugar. So artificial sweeteners only trick the brain into craving more sweets and more sugar and throw your blood sugar levels out of balance. Also, our bodies weren't designed to process artificial ingredients. When you ingest these, the body can't figure out what to do with them. So it surrounds these mystery chemicals with fat and tucks them away someplace you'd probably rather they'd not be. So even though that diet soda you sip doesn't technically hurt your calorie intake, it does no favors to your body.

Junk Food

Just about anything that comes in a box (with the exception of whole grains) or enveloped in a candy wrapper is junk food. It's normally loaded with sugar, trans fats, and preservatives. If you eat more sugar than you burn off, your body generates fat. Globs of sunny yellow fat—unused glucose that's now turned to fat—float in your blood through your arteries to the organ or tissues where they are deposited. When fat finds a home somewhere, you get fat and look fat. That's the cosmetic problem we all hate and want to do away with. Also critical: when fat homesteads in an organ, it can cause big problems, from heart disease to diabetes to outright organ failure. So, junk the junk.

Fast Food

Watch fast-food restaurants, too. Sure, I like a good drive-through burger as much as the next guy. And I'll allow myself a couple of them a year, but that's it. I know people though who eat fast food several times a week, if not every day, and slam down soda like the fountain is about to run dry. Our spiraling weight problems are a product of a society obsessed with fast and convenient food. When we're in a hurry and want to eat, those cheeseburgers and fries seem much more appealing than a salad.

They can be addictive, too. Scientists at Rockefeller University in New York discovered that fast food, with all its hidden fat and sugar, can spark druglike chemical reactions in the brain that can make you overeat. These reactions are comparable to those triggered by taking drugs such as heroin and cocaine. So if you're serious about getting in peak shape, don't grace the doors of too many fast-food joints.

Every time you eat any food, whether it's a piece of cheesecake, a cut of beef, or a leafy green salad, your body will use it for energy or store it as fat. You have the power to control whether that food is burned (along with stored body fat) or packed away as unsightly fat. The way you switch your body from fat storing to fat burning is by eating real fuel from the Magnificent 7 and shifting calories up and down in a systemic fashion.

Within a few weeks of eating like this, you'll have adapted to a livable, sustainable way of eating and exercising, and I doubt if you'll lapse back into any bad fat-gaining habits. When you can say "I love this diet!" then you're on your way to a trimmer, fitter, more attractive you.

CHAPTER 5

BLOCK OUT FAT-BURNING, MUSCLE-BUILDING NUTRITION

You'll eat all of the Magnificent 7 foods according to meal patterns I call "blocks." There are three blocks in this diet, deliberately designed to help you steadily lose unwanted weight, week by week. As you move through the blocks, you'll be motivated to continue right down to your ideal goal because you'll constantly be shedding weight. You'll immediately begin to feel better, too, because you'll be giving your body exactly what it wants and needs.

The three blocks are based on calorie cycling (variations in calories). Remember, though, you don't have to count any calories, or calculate grams of macronutrients. Rather, I'll give you defined servings for all meals and snacks, so all you need to do is select the right foods and/or follow the meal plans. As you move from Block 3 to Block 2 to Block 1, you'll be naturally eating a little less, but because the meal plans are designed with a variety of food suggestions, you'll feel satisfied.

The three blocks are so simple that you have virtually nothing to memorize. Each meal is organized into a pattern, which is basically a recommended combination of protein and carbohydrates. You'll get ample fat from protein, plant sources such as nuts and seeds, and optional oils such as coconut or olive oil.

The portion sizes are standardized for men and women so that once you understand and practice them, you'll be able to eventually eyeball the amounts without weighing or measuring. You'll be able to do the plan anywhere you go or travel.

BLOCK 3

Block 3 lasts for three weeks. In this block, you'll be eating four fast-fuel carbs daily. The overall goal of Block 3 is to introduce you to the Magnificent 7 foods and start the fat-burning, muscle-building process.

Here's what Block 3 looks like.

Block 3 Carbs

Your daily carb allotment is four fast-fuel carbs and a liberal amount of slow-fuel carbs.

Breakfast Pattern:

Protein + 1 serving fast-fuel carb.

BREAKFAST EXAMPLES

1 PROTEIN	1 FAST-FUEL CARB	BONUS FUELS/ CONDIMENTS
2 scrambled eggs	1 serving (cooked) instant oatmeal	1 teaspoon honey, if desired
2 turkey sausages	1 slice whole-grain or sprouted-grain toast	All-fruit jam for your toast, if desired
*Smoothie: 1 serving vegetable-based protein powder	¼ cup (uncooked) instant oatmeal	1 tablespoon coconut oil + 1 cup almond milk

* Feel free to add a fruit to your smoothie; just count it as one of your fast-fuel carbs for the day.

Lunch Pattern:

Protein + 1 serving fast-fuel carb and liberal amounts of slow-fuel carbs.

LUNCH EXAMPLES

1 PROTEIN	1 FAST-FUEL CARB	SLOW-FUEL CARBS	BONUS FUELS/ CONDIMENTS
1 grilled chicken breast	1 serving brown rice	1 tossed salad	(1–2 tablespoons low-fat salad dressing)
Tuna	Apple	1 tossed salad	(1–2 tablespoons low-fat salad dressing)
Lean ground beef	1 serving kidney beans	Chopped green pepper	Made into chili using tomato sauce and spices

Dinner Pattern:

Protein + 1 serving fast-fuel carb and liberal amounts of slow-fuel carbs.

DINNER EXAMPLES

1 PROTEIN	1 FAST-FUEL CARB	SLOW-FUEL CARBS	BONUS FUELS/ CONDIMENTS
Grilled rib-eye steak	Baked sweet potato	Steamed green beans	Steak sauce
Baked salmon	Winter squash	Steamed broccoli	Herbs and spices
Baked or grilled chicken thighs	1 serving brown rice	Stir-fried vegetables	1–2 tablespoons olive oil for stir-frying

***Snack Pattern* (1 midmorning, 1 midafternoon):**

Protein + nuts or seeds or a slow-fuel vegetable, or after your workout, a protein + a fast-fuel carb.

SNACK EXAMPLES

1 PROTEIN	1 FAST-FUEL CARB	SLOW-FUEL CARB/FAT FUEL/BONUS FUELS/ CONDIMENTS
1–2 hard-boiled eggs		Handful of raw almonds
½ grilled chicken breast	1 slice sprouted-grain bread	
*Smoothie: 1 serving vegetable-based protein powder	¼ cup (uncooked) instant oatmeal, or 1 fruit serving	Handful of spinach, 1 tablespoon coconut oil + 1 cup almond milk

* Feel free to add a fruit to your smoothie; just count it as one of your fast-fuel carbs for the day.

Guidelines for Block 3

1. Follow your daily carb allotment: 4 fast-fuel carbs at meals or snacks, and as many slow-fuel carbs as you want.
2. Use the meal patterns as a guideline to help structure your meals.
3. Vary your food selections, and use my recipes.
4. Don't skip snacks or meals, especially breakfast, in order to control possible cravings.
5. Eat until you're satisfied but not stuffed.
6. Stay well hydrated.
7. Stay on Block 3 for three weeks.

BLOCK 2

Block 2 starts at week 4. In this block, you start cycling down your calories and carbs by reducing your servings of fast-fuel carbs from four servings to two servings a day. Thus, your daily carb allotment is two fast-fuel carbs daily and liberal servings of slow-fuel carbs.

Breakfast Pattern:

Protein + 1 fast-fuel carb = ideal Body Fuel breakfast for Block 2.

BREAKFAST EXAMPLES

1 PROTEIN	1 FAST-FUEL CARB	BONUS FUELS/ CONDIMENTS
2 slices Canadian bacon	1 serving packaged cereal (corn flakes, high-fiber cereal, or an enriched cereal such as Special K or Total)	1 cup almond milk (bonus fuel) for the cereal
2 turkey sausages	1 slice whole-grain or sprouted-grain toast	All-fruit jam for your toast, if desired
Smoothie: 1 serving vegetable-based protein powder	1 banana	1 tablespoon coconut oil + 1 cup almond milk

Lunch Pattern:

Protein + 1 fast-fuel carb + slow-fuel carbs = ideal Body Fuel lunch for Block 2.

LUNCH EXAMPLES

1 PROTEIN	1 FAST-FUEL CARB	SLOW-FUEL CARBS	BONUS FUELS/ CONDIMENTS
1 grilled chicken breast	1 serving brown rice	1 tossed salad	(1–2 tablespoons low-fat salad dressing)
Tuna	1 slice sprouted-grain bread	Tomato slices and alfalfa sprouts to top the sandwich	(1–2 tablespoons low-fat mayonnaise to mix with the tuna)
Lean ground beef	1 serving kidney beans	Chopped green pepper	Made into chili using tomato sauce and spices

Dinner Pattern:

Protein + slow-fuel carbs = ideal Body Fuel dinner for Block 2.

DINNER EXAMPLES

1 PROTEIN	SLOW-FUEL CARBS	BONUS FUELS/ CONDIMENTS
Grilled pork chop	Steamed yellow squash and spinach	Teriyaki sauce
Roast turkey breast	Steamed broccoli and cauliflower	Herbs and spices
Lean ground beef	Zucchini strips	No-sugar-added marinara sauce, cooked with lean ground beef and poured over zucchini strips

***Snack Pattern* (1 midmorning, 1 midafternoon):**

Protein + nuts or seeds or a non-starchy vegetable, or a post-workout fast-fuel carb (if not eaten at one of your three main meals) = ideal snack for Block 2.

SNACK EXAMPLES

1 PROTEIN	1 FAST-FUEL CARB	SLOW-FUEL CARB/FAT FUEL/BONUS FUELS/ CONDIMENTS
1–2 hard-boiled eggs		Handful of raw almonds
½ grilled chicken breast	Raw non-starchy vegetable sticks	
Smoothie: 1 serving vegetable-based protein powder	¼ cup (uncooked) instant oatmeal	Handful of spinach, 1 tablespoon coconut oil + 1 cup almond milk

Guidelines for Block 2

1. Follow your daily carb allotment: two fast-fuel carbs at meals or snacks, and as many slow-fuel carbs as you want.
2. Use the meal patterns as a guideline to help structure your meals.
3. Vary your food selections, and use my recipes.
4. Don't skip snacks or meals, especially breakfast.
5. Eat until you're satisfied but not stuffed.
6. Stay well hydrated.
7. Stay on Block 2 for two weeks.

BLOCK 1

Begin Block 1 at week 5. In this block, you further cycle down your calories and carbs. Your daily carb allotment is one fast-fuel carb, eaten for breakfast or after your workout, and as many slow-fuel carbs as you want.

Breakfast Pattern:

Protein + 1 fast-fuel carb or 1 slow-fuel carb = ideal Body Fuel breakfast for Block 1.

BREAKFAST EXAMPLES

1 PROTEIN	1 FAST-FUEL CARB/AND 1 SLOW-FUEL CARB, IF DESIRED	BONUS FUELS/ CONDIMENTS
2 poached eggs	½ grapefruit	Cinnamon on grapefruit
2 turkey sausages	1 slice whole-grain or sprouted-grain toast	All-fruit jam for your toast, if desired
Smoothie: 1 serving vegetable-based protein powder	1 cup berries	1 tablespoon coconut oil + 1 cup almond milk

Lunch Pattern:

Protein + slow-fuel vegetable = ideal Body Fuel lunch for Block 1.

LUNCH EXAMPLES

1 PROTEIN	SLOW-FUEL CARBS	BONUS FUELS/ CONDIMENTS
Grilled chicken breast	Romaine lettuce and other salad veggies	1–2 tablespoons low-fat salad dressing
Boiled shrimp	Sliced cucumbers	Herbs and spices
Tuna	Lettuce and other salad veggies	1–2 tablespoons low-fat salad dressing

Dinner Pattern:

Protein + slow-fuel non-starchy vegetable = ideal Body Fuel dinner for Block 1.

DINNER EXAMPLES

1 PROTEIN	SLOW-FUEL CARBS	BONUS FUELS/ CONDIMENTS
Prime rib	Mashed cauliflower and cooked green beans	Herbs and spices
Baked tilapia	Cooked zucchini	Herbs and spices
Lean ground beef patty	Baked eggplant slices and tossed salad	No-sugar-added marinara sauce to top the eggplant; 1–2 tablespoons low-fat salad dressing

SNACK EXAMPLES

1 PROTEIN	1 SLOW-FUEL CARB	FAT FUEL/BONUS FUELS/CONDIMENTS
1–2 hard-boiled eggs		Handful of raw almonds
½ grilled chicken breast	Fresh vegetable juice	
Smoothie: 1 serving vegetable-based protein powder	Handful of spinach	1 tablespoon coconut oil + 1 cup almond milk

Guidelines for Block 1

1. Follow your daily carb allotment: one fast-fuel carb at a meal or as a post-workout snack, and as many slow-fuel carbs as you want.
2. Use the meal patterns as a guideline to help structure your meals.
3. Vary your food selections, and use my recipes.
4. Don't skip snacks or meals, especially breakfast.
5. Eat until you're satisfied but not stuffed.

6. Stay well hydrated.
7. Stay on Block 1 for one week.
8. Afterward, repeat the Body Fuel calorie cycling: Block 3 for three weeks, Block 2 for two weeks, and Block 1 for one week. Keep repeating my calorie-cycling method until you reach your ideal weight.

IF YOU NEED TO GAIN WEIGHT

Many people wish they had your problem. For them, gaining weight is easy. However, for some people—even athletes—gaining weight is tough. To put on quality weight (muscle), you must take in more calories than you expend.

The first step to gaining weight is to eat extra calories each day—between 500 and 1,000 additional calories daily—at least until a weight gain occurs. To put on one pound of muscle, it takes an additional 27.2 calories per pound of body weight. So if you're a tall guy, say six feet, and you weigh only 150 pounds, that means you'd have to eat at least 4,080 calories a day.

Toward this end, stay on Block 3 only. This keeps you on a schedule of eating three main meals a day and at least two snacks. To increase your calories, drink a high-calorie smoothie between meals as your snack. That's a good way to easily ingest many extra calories, and always have a fast-fuel carb after your workouts. You're going to have to eat like it's a second job, which is exactly what it can feel like. This will ensure that you are replenishing muscle glycogen and storing it, so that your muscles stay in an anabolic state.

Speaking of protein, make sure you have protein at every meal and snack. For weight gain, figure on eating up to 1.5 grams of protein per pound of your body weight. Protein is essential for putting on muscle.

Another piece of advice is to increase your daily calories by incorporating one of my high-calorie smoothies in your daily diet. You can find the recipes starting on page 121.

As for workouts, stay consistent, and do mostly resistance training in order to gain muscle mass.

Keep a close eye on your body composition—the relative proportion of muscle to body fat. If you notice yourself packing on more fat than you feel comfortable with, switch to Block 2 until you get that fat off. On the other hand, if you're not seeing any changes, return to Block 3 and bump up your calories even more by eating more protein, adding an extra snack, or including one or two additional servings of fast-fuel carbs to your daily intake.

Keep in mind that if you're trying to build serious muscle mass, it's inevitable you'll pack on a little body fat at the same time. Don't worry about it too much. Focus on eating enough and gaining strength. Then, after you've got your muscle, shift your focus to losing body fat to show them off. Going on Block 2 or even Block 1 will help you accomplish this.

Gaining quality weight can be easier than you think if you do all the right things: eat high-protein meals, enjoy plenty of quality fast-fuel and slow-fuel carbs, have frequent meals, and work out intensely. Do all this, and you'll find gaining muscle a rewarding endeavor.

A QUICK AND EASY OVERVIEW OF THE BODY FUEL PLAN

BLOCK 3 (3 WEEKS): 4 FAST-FUEL CARBS DAILY AND LIBERAL AMOUNTS OF SLOW-FUEL CARBS	
BREAKFAST	Protein + 1 fast-fuel carb
LUNCH	Protein + 1 fast-fuel carb + slow-fuel carbs
DINNER	Protein + 1 fast-fuel carb + slow-fuel carbs
SNACK 1	Protein + 1 fast-fuel carb
SNACK 2	Protein + slow-fuel carbs
BLOCK 2 (2 WEEKS): 2 FAST-FUEL CARBS DAILY AND LIBERAL AMOUNTS OF SLOW-FUEL CARBS	
BREAKFAST	Protein + 1 fast-fuel carb
LUNCH	Protein + 1 fast-fuel carb + slow-fuel carbs
DINNER	Protein + slow-fuel carbs
SNACK 1	Protein + slow-fuel carbs
SNACK 2	Protein + slow-fuel carbs (or one of your fast-fuel carbs if taken after your workout)

BLOCK 1 (1 WEEK): 1 FAST-FUEL CARB DAILY AND LIBERAL AMOUNTS OF SLOW-FUEL CARBS	
BREAKFAST	Protein + 1 fast-fuel carb
LUNCH	Protein + slow-fuel carbs
DINNER	Protein + slow-fuel carbs
SNACK 1	Protein + slow-fuel carbs
SNACK 2	Protein + slow-fuel carbs (or your fast-fuel carb if taken after your workout)

As you go through the blocks, don't give in to the temptation of not eating, skipping meals, or overexercising—all of which can cause muscle loss and counteract your goals. You must do everything in your power to prevent muscle loss while losing weight. Remember, it isn't simply about losing weight. It's about body composition—less fat and more lean muscle. Follow all three blocks, and you'll succeed.

CHAPTER 6

ZERO WEEK—FALL IN!

I want you to feel that you're truly ready for this program—not just that you "should" do it, but that you have an inner resolve to get in shape and stay there, and you know the time is now. Have you thought hard about those Marked Foods that you might be willing to give up for a while, for example? What foods to eat more of? Whether, if you eat out a lot, you're willing to stop overindulging at restaurants? Have you already tried any particular healthful lifestyle steps to see if you can live with them? Have you carefully considered the difference between wanting something and being prepared to pay a price for whatever you want?

Moving into a state of total readiness is something I compare to "Zero Week" in the military. Zero Week is thus named so that some of the tougher schools can boast quick "four-week" training courses, when in fact the courses are longer. I remember when I showed up for the Army's Special Forces Dive School in Key West, Florida, where the military's elite train at some of the most physically demanding tasks in the military. I was told that it would be only a four-week school. Man, was I disheartened after I found out it would actually be five weeks.

The first week was Zero Week. The instructors put us through a grueling series of tests conducted in a swimming pool. One of the tests required that we swim underwater for fifty meters on just a single breath. You aren't allowed to touch any part of the pool or even come up for air. The toughest test, though, was drownproofing. Instructors bound our hands and feet with Velcro straps and plopped us in the water. We had to bob up and down in deep water until told to stop. If we broke the straps or touched the sides of the pool, we'd fail. The whole time I was thinking, "What did I get myself into?"

Zero Week was designed to weed out people who weren't meant to be combat divers. The course itself was one of the hardest I've ever completed. I'm glad I did it, but I was also glad when it was over.

I want you to start my program with a Zero Week. Don't freak out—you won't be required to swim underwater or bob up and down with your hands and feet bound! But you can use this same concept to get a better start on your diet, and of course with the intent of making things as easy as possible.

My Zero Week is a time to get down to business, stretch yourself in certain areas, and discover that you're capable of more than you ever thought possible. I want you to methodically get ready, mentally and physically, for the upcoming wholesale change you'll be making in your eating habits.

Zero Week is about making baby steps. In my work with people all over the world, I've found that slow baby steps are the best ways to prepare and, ultimately, to change. So don't wing it unprepared. You wouldn't go on a road trip or plan a new business strategy without advanced preparation. Why tackle one of the most important health moves you'll be taking without giving it just as much—if not more—thought and attention?

Zero Week starts now. Take the following steps this week:

DAY 1: STOP DRINKING YOUR CALORIES

After embarking on a weight loss diet, it's logical to rethink what you put on your plate. But it's just as important to rethink what you're pouring into a glass or a mug. Liquid calories can be worse than solid food when it comes to weight gain. By liquid calories, I mean soft drinks or soda, as well as alcoholic beverages, fruity drinks, punches, and any high-calorie beverage sweetened with sugar. Soda is particularly bad, and one of the beverages making people fat. A single can of soda per day can add up to about fifteen pounds of fat over the course of a year. Soda is the largest source of sugar in our diets, delivering a third of all added sugars.

Scientific proof is piling up that our bodies don't register the calories in liquids the same way as when we eat solid foods. In fact, a 2008 study published in *Obesity Reviews* suggested that in terms of appetite regulation, the body hormonally acknowledges fluids differently than it does solid foods. The problem is that liquids don't subdue ghrelin—the body's hunger-stimulating hormone—as well as solid foods do. Consequently, you may still feel hungry even after you've had something to drink. Without the appropriate appetite-control signals kicking in, you may overeat and thus consume more calories. This happened in the landmark Nurses' Health Study, which tracked more than fifty thousand women for eight years. The study found that women who cut back on their intake of sugar-sweetened beverages were able to automatically reduce calories by an average of 319 a day—and were thus able to lose weight. Other women who upped their consumption of sugary beverages from one drink a week to one or more a day consumed an extra 358 calories a day, and they *gained* weight.

So today, think before you drink. Some suggestions:

- Cut out all sodas—diet and otherwise.
- Drink more water: tap (filtered tap is best to remove chemicals and impurities), bottled, or sparkling. Make it tastier by adding some lemon or lime juice or a few cucumber slices. Shoot for 8 cups of water daily at a minimum.

- If you decide to juice, make it vegetable juice mainly, around 8 to 10 ounces per serving.
- As for fruit juice, don't drink it. You'll take in too many sugary calories, and you'll be unable to fully tame cravings for sweets.
- Enjoy certain herbal teas. These are a terrific way to get some extra fluid into your system. You'll get extra nutrients and health protection, too. Chamomile tea, for example, has anti-germ and anti-clotting properties. Peppermint tea has antiviral, antioxidant, and antitumor properties. And green tea packs in more antioxidants than many vegetables do.
- Beware of specialty waters, which are not always calorie-free these days and might contain artificial sweeteners.
- Drink alcohol in moderation this week if you drink at all. That means one alcoholic beverage a day for women, two for men. More than that, and you may invite health and accident risks into your life. Also, calories from overimbibing wine, beer, and cocktails add up fast.

Zero Week Daily Checklist

Today:

✔ I cut out liquid calories.

DAY 2: EAT ONE RAW GREEN SALAD A DAY

One of the healthiest dishes ever, green salads not only help you lose fat and inches but also keep many lifestyle diseases at bay. This is because salads are generally made with leafy vegetables, such as romaine and other lettuces, spinach, arugula, kale, bok choy, cabbage, and Swiss chard. All are true superfoods that have been credited with everything from better heart health to protection from bone-crippling osteoporosis. Leafy greens are low in calories and rich in fiber, making them perfect for weight control. Plus they're potent sources of phytonutrients, vitamins, and minerals. What's not to love about these leafy superfoods?

When you add a salad as a first course to your meal, you'll automatically trim calories from your bottom line. Pennsylvania State University researchers found that starting lunch with a healthful salad (3 cups' worth) reduced the total number of calories volunteers ate at the meal (and the main meal was easy-to-fill-up-on pasta!).

Here's how to apply all these great facts to Zero Week:

- Have a large salad (about 2 to 3 cups of greens and salad veggies) as a first course for either lunch or dinner. Do this daily, and you'll get a burst of slow-fuel carbs into your body.
- Use a lot of different types of greens to build your salads. That way, you'll take advantage of all the nutrient power green leafy vegetables provide.
- Watch out for add-ons, such as croutons, bacon bits, nuts, cheese, and creamy dressings. If you eat all that on a salad, you might as well have a cheeseburger (don't even think about it!).
- Perk up your salad with a tablespoon or two of low-fat or nonfat salad dressings, or better yet, go to MarkLauren.com for some great homemade salad dressings.
- Vary your salads and the greens you use as a base. Try a spinach salad, for example.
- Make a main course salad: pile on some greens and salad veggies, add some tuna or lean meat, cooked black beans or corn, and toss with nonfat salad dressing.

Zero Week Daily Checklist

Today:

✔ I cut out liquid calories.

✔ I ate one salad.

DAY 3: PLAN YOUR FIRST WEEK'S MENU

It's easier to lose weight and stay in shape when you have a good plan. Without a plan, forget it. Meal planning gives you control over what you eat, takes the guesswork out of meals, and helps you avoid spontaneous, out-of-control indulgences in unhealthful food choices.

Doing so may even double your weight loss, too. A 2008 study of seventeen hundred overweight people published in the *American Journal of Preventive Medicine* showed that dieters who consistently recorded their food intake lost double the pounds of those who kept no records over the course of twenty weeks.

Start this habit today. Sit down and write out your meals and snacks for week 1. There are a few easy ways to approach this:

- Skip ahead to page 80 and read through the suggested meal plan for week 1 of Block 3. You have the option to follow this meal plan exactly as it is, if desired. A lot of people prefer to follow a set meal plan because it removes guesswork from the eating equation. A set meal plan also helps you become accustomed to the diet.
- Another option is to plan out your own meals using my Body Fuel guidelines. There's a meal planning template you can use in the Appendix (page 235). The more detailed you can be, the better results you'll have—a fact that's backed up by science. Researchers at Brown University's Weight Control and Diabetes Research Center in Providence, Rhode Island, observed what happened when two groups of women kept food diaries. One group kept very detailed records of what they ate; the other group kept fewer details. They women who were more detailed in their diaries lost twice as much weight as those who kept shorter, less detailed diaries.
- Choose a combination of my two meal planning tips. You might follow my meals exactly on some days. On others, you might plan your own. This method gives you some structure along with flexibility. My meals plans are as adaptable as you want to make them.

Just remember that creating meal plans and writing them down is a proven, validated method of keeping tabs on your food consumption and modifying your eating behavior.

Zero Week Daily Checklist

Today:

✔ I cut out liquid calories.

✔ I ate one salad.

✔ I wrote out my meal plan in detail for week 1, Block 3.

DAY 4: DO A KITCHEN CLEANOUT

Here's where I want you to toss out all junk food from your pantry and fridge. Unless you change what's in your cupboards, the chances are you'll find temptation catching up with you sooner or later.

Check labels and toss out anything that contains high-fructose corn syrup, added sugar in any form, hydrogenated oils (trans fats), artificial flavors, dyes and colorings, preservatives, and other questionable or hard-to-pronounce chemicals. These will include foods like cookies, chips, and snack foods.

While you're at it:

- Check "best by" dates on all packaged foods. Get rid of anything that may have expired or items that you hardly use and are nearing their expiration date.
- For hygienic purposes and to protect your food, wipe down surfaces. Before restocking, clean shelving with a food-safe, gentle cleanser to eliminate any dirt, germs, and so forth.

Out of sight, out of mouth: you may be able to shed a couple of pounds during Zero Week simply by cleaning out your kitchen and thus steering clear of fattening junk food.

Zero Week Daily Checklist

Today:

✔ I cut out liquid calories.

✔ I ate one salad.

✔ I have my meal plan ready for week 1, Block 3.

✔ I did a kitchen cleanout—and will keep junk food out of my home.

DAY 5: WRITE DOWN YOUR GOALS

At the beginning of each year, then again at midyear, I write out my goals for what I want to achieve, from future income streams to physical achievements. Failing to set goals is a common mistake. I don't want you to make that mistake, so let's do some goal setting right now.

- Set your goals with the end in mind. In the military, mission planning is done with a "backward-planning" timeline. You start with actions on the objective and plan backward from that point after thoroughly establishing what the objective is, what criteria must be met for mission success, and how they will be achieved. Then execution is simply a matter of not giving up. You already have in this book a sound nutritional plan, along with a workout, that will get you in the best shape of your life. It is much easier to achieve any goal if you have a clear picture of the goal. Have a vision of what you want to look like. One way to do this is to find a picture of a physically fit person who has a body type similar to yours. Imagine yourself looking like that person. So identify the end you have in mind. Eating properly and consistently working out will get you there.
- Be specific. Your goal may be to get fitter, lose weight, exercise more, or eat healthier, but that's far too vague. You've got to zero in, with detail, creating goals that are measurable and realistic. Take the goal of losing weight, for example. Decide exactly how many pounds you

want to lose, and set a timeline (how long it will take) and a target date for that weight loss. If you want to increase exercise frequency, decide how many times a week you want to work out. Setting specific and measurable goals keeps you motivated and allows you to assess your progress along the way.

- Devise actionable strategies daily. When it comes down to achieving your goals, it's about the consistent, daily actions you take each day. Those actions are really mini-goals that get you to your big goals. Examples of mini-goals are: *I will eat three to five servings of slow-fuel carbs today. I will drink 8 cups of water today. I will work out today.* So plan your day before it begins. Chunk your major goals into actionable steps and activities. Write these down each day—and follow through. Those mini-goals will keep you from feeling overwhelmed because as you complete them, you'll immediately see your progress. I like to write my to-do lists at night before going to sleep.
- Identify your excuses and find solutions. We all create excuses, all the time, to blow off our diets or our workouts. So often, excuses become more important than the goals you've set for yourself. Excuses I've heard include:

    - *Eating healthfully is too much trouble.*
    - *I don't have the energy.*
    - *Vegetables taste boring.*
    - *I can't control my cravings.*
    - *I don't feel like it.*
    - *I'll start tomorrow, or next week.*

Of course, all of these are complete nonsense, and they will keep you from reaching your goals if you buy into them. My advice is to write down your excuses, then come up with strategies to counteract them. For example, if you don't have time to exercise, create a strategy such as scheduling your workout on your calendar like you would any appointment—then keeping it. Remember, too, that my workouts are time-efficient. I mean, who can't find the time to work out for twenty to thirty minutes at least three times a week? You can do my workouts anywhere! Or, if you have trouble with vegetables, commit to trying something new, such as roasting them in the oven with a little olive oil and herbs. If bad moods and stress are excuses to overeat, work on relaxation techniques. For every excuse, there's a solution!

You must absolutely write down your goals, daily actions, and excuses. Doing so is a small sacrifice to make in order to gain a long, healthy, and fit life.

Zero Week Daily Checklist

Today:

✔ I cut out liquid calories.

✔ I ate one salad.

✔ I have my meal plan ready for week 1, Block 3.

✔ I kept junk food out of my home.

✔ I wrote down my goals.

DAY 6: SHOP AND PREP

With your meal plan in hand, create a shopping list of the foods you'll need for your first week. Don't forget items such as recommended condiments and bonus fuels. Most of these can be purchased at your local grocery store. Stock up on fresh herbs such as ginger, green onions, and cilantro, too. These really perk up meals all on their own. Try to buy organic foods whenever possible in order to cut down on chemicals, preservatives, hormones, and pesticides. Stick to your list.

Next, begin to develop a weekend ritual in which you not only shop, but also prepare and package a good portion of your week's food. I recommend meal prepping right after shopping, if possible. Once you put everything in the fridge, you might forget to prep or have an excuse to skip it.

When you prep, many of your meals can be "grab and go." Even though this ritual of making meals in advance requires a little extra effort, it will save you an incredible amount of time, money, and joy lost to preventable illnesses. If you think preparing your own food is inconvenient, consider the inconvenience of having diabetes, heart disease, or cancer.

Here are my suggestions for mapping out a convenient week of eating:

- Have carrots and other salad veggies peeled and cut up, ready for your salads.
- As a timesaver, purchase precut lettuces and salad veggies to prepare your salads. Or stop by the supermarket and scoop up your salad from its salad bar.
- Make your salad ahead of time, too. Layer your salad ingredients in a deep plastic container. Always place the cooked meat on the bottom of the container, because the meat juice or the weight will cause the veggies to brown. Then stack your vegetables, from the heaviest to the lightest: cucumbers, carrots, lettuce, and so forth. I usually make my own dressing (see the recipe section). Then I put some in a zip-top bag and place it at the top of the container and close the lid. This procedure makes an easy grab-and-go salad.
- Right after grocery shopping, marinate all of your meats with fresh or dry herbs and seasonings. Doing so locks in the flavor.
- Grill, bake, or otherwise cook all of your meat for the first half of the week. Package the remaining uncooked meat in serving sizes and freeze it. This way it's easy to use only what you need. Then, midweek, thaw more meat and cook it for the rest of the week. Pack any cooked meat in a container. Use separate containers for different types of meats.
- After shopping, wash and cut up all of your veggies. Then cook up large batches and refrigerate them. Warm them up in your microwave for meals. You can do the same with frozen vegetables.
- Bake your potatoes, sweet potatoes, and yams in bulk, then store them in a large container. If you don't have time to bake, I would wash the potatoes, pierce them, and microwave them on high, 5 minutes per potato.
- Plan your snacks. Package single servings of nuts, veggies, and fruits

in zip-top bags. Take them with you while running errands. This will prevent the urge to swing by fast-food restaurants if you're hungry, or keep you from falling victim to food billboards or signs that make your mouth water.

- Get into cooking. Cooking can be daunting if you're new to it, but like anything else, practice makes perfect. With more experience, you'll cut in half the amount of time you need to spend cooking and be able to tweak my recipes to suit your specific tastes. Don't be scared to make mistakes and experiment. A little trial and error goes a long way. This isn't life or death; after all, you're not calling in air strikes. It's okay to learn from your mistakes.

With a little practice, preparing and cooking food this way will become second nature.

Zero Week Daily Checklist

Today:

✔ I cut out liquid calories.

✔ I ate one salad.

✔ I have my meal plan ready for week 1, Block 3.

✔ I kept junk food out of my home.

✔ I reviewed my goals.

✔ I shopped for the right foods—and prepped them.

Hoo-ya!

Locally Grown and Raised Is Often the Cheapest and Healthiest

Healthwise, it's important to consider the methods used to grow or raise our food and also the process used to get that food into our hands. When it comes to cost, nutritional value, and taste, shorter food chains are superior to longer ones. And the grub with the shortest food chains is found at your local farmer's market, where you get to interact directly with the people in your community who are growing your food.

By contrast, most food in the United States travels an average of 1,500 miles to get to your dinner table, according to the Center for Urban Education about Sustainable Agriculture, a nonprofit organization dedicated to promoting an environmentally friendly food system. All of this transportation uses up fuel, contributes to pollution, and creates excess trash due to packaging. Food at the farmer's market is transported shorter distances, thus minimizing environmental impact.

What's more, the produce you buy at your local farmer's market is fresher and tastier than what you get in your grocery store. Plus, a lot of food from grocery stores is grown using pesticides, hormones, antibiotics, and genetic modification—all practices that may harm your health. You're less likely to find adulterated food from your local farmers, who tend to produce food using sustainable, and often organic, methods. The food tends to be less expensive, too, than many foods at the grocery store.

If you haven't already, give your local farmer's market or Asian market a try. Both offer a huge variety of fruits and vegetables grown locally. Even if it doesn't become a regular thing, it's a good educational experience to know what your options are. Plus, these markets can be far cheaper than buying organic produce at a supermarket.

DAY 7: FAST!

This might be the most challenging day in Zero Week. It's the last day, and I want you to fast, at least from dinner one day to dinner the next.

By "fasting," I mean abstaining from most foods. Fasting is commonly observed in religious traditions, spiritual practices, self-control exercises, and health programs.

In addition to temporarily reducing your caloric intake, fasting grants your body an opportunity to cleanse itself internally and to detoxify from exposures to environmental pollutants and our daily ingestion of processed and refined foods.

I'm recommending a one-day fast only—to get you primed to start Block 3. Even after one day of fasting, you may:

- Utilize more body fat for energy
- Sharpen your senses and feel revitalized
- Have reduced cravings for your usual sugary or fatty foods
- Realize that it's okay to feel hungry—that hunger is mostly psychological anyway, a response triggered by time of day, your routine, or smells of food
- Experience self-discipline to help you feel empowered throughout the entire program

During this one-day fast:

- Drink 8 to 10 cups of water throughout the day. It's fine to enjoy herbal tea as well. Drinking plenty of fluids helps move toxins through your urinary system and prevent constipation.
- Have "fasting food," if you feel very hungry. By this, I mean some green vegetables, preferably raw, such as lettuce, celery, cucumbers, or various greens.
- Don't exercise, so that you can conserve energy. Instead, rest by pampering yourself, watching videos, or listening to music—and expect to feel energetic and look better the following week.

- Plan your fast for the weekend, preferably Sunday, when your activities are minimized and you can keep things as stress-free as possible.
- If you feel light-headed, dizzy, or otherwise not normal, stop the fast by drinking some vegetable juice and eating some light foods such as a salad.

Fasting can be a great instrument for weight control, health, and self-discipline. You might consider setting aside a fast day between each block of the program, too.

Zero Week Daily Checklist

Today:

✔ I cut out liquid calories.

✔ I ate one salad.

✔ I have my meal plan ready for week 1, Block 3.

✔ I kept junk food out of my home.

✔ I reviewed my goals.

✔ I shopped for the right foods—and prepped them.

✔ I fasted.

I hope Zero Week has been fun and educational for you, a time to ease into a new way of living. From here, it's time to build an awareness of what you put in your body, and apply my nutritional strategies to reach and sustain your fitness goals.

I hereby declare Zero Week over . . . you're good to go!

PART 3

POWER UP

CHAPTER 7

YOU ARE YOUR OWN NUTRITIONIST: THE BODY FUEL MEAL PLANS

Most of you have probably followed meal plans from other diets in the past and made a pledge to stick to them until you are trim and fit again. But at some point you didn't get to that goal. Anyone who fits that category, please step forward. It's time to put an end to failure and take control of your own diet.

With Body Fuel, I'm giving you six weeks of sample meals to illustrate how the blocks work in real life. These meal plans represent a template demonstrating how fast fuels and slow fuels can be arranged during the different blocks to help you achieve the metabolic benefits of calorie cycling. It is an easily followed plan, and you can do it to the letter, down to the very last snack. However, I want you to learn to be your own nutritionist, tweak the plan, and work it around your own goals, metabolism, gender, and activity levels, not anyone else's. The plan is intentionally flexible and meant to be customized to best suit individual needs.

Let's talk about how to do that.

HOW MUCH FOOD SHOULD YOU EAT?

The amount of food that constitutes the right portion for you boils down to hands, fingers, and thumbs. In other words, a good, easy-to-use measurement of what constitutes a serving of protein, fast fuel, slow fuel, or fat is to see if it fits in the palm of your hand or matches the size of your finger or thumb.

Protein

If you're a man, you're going to require a larger quantity of protein, anywhere from 6 to 8 ounces at lunch and dinner, while a woman needs 3 to 5 ounces. So basically, the amount of protein you can fit in the palm of your hand automatically gives you the correct amount for your gender. For other proteins that don't measure well by the hand method, refer to the following chart:

FOOD	MEN'S SERVING SIZE	WOMEN'S SERVING SIZE
Eggs	3–4	2
Egg whites	4–6	3–4
Egg substitute	1 cup	½ cup
Plant-based protein (beans and legumes)	1 cup	½ cup
Protein powders	1–2 scoops	1 scoop
Protein bars	1 bar	1 bar
Shellfish (shrimp, oysters, scallops, etc.)	2 cups	1 cup

Fast Fuels

A portion of a fast fuel such as a grain, cereal, pasta, legumes, or berries should be no bigger than your fist when clenched. A fruit portion is typically a single piece of fruit. Some other helpful measurements for men and women are listed below:

FOOD	MEN'S SERVING SIZE	WOMEN'S SERVING SIZE
Grains (rice, couscous, oatmeal, grits, barley, quinoa, etc.)	1 cup	½ cup
Ready-to-eat cereal	1 cup to 1¼ cups (read package instructions for exact measurement)	1 cup to 1¼ cups (read package instructions for exact measurement)
Pasta	1 cup	½ cup
Plant-based protein (beans and legumes)	1 cup	½ cup
Starchy vegetables (beets, carrots, corn, parsnips, peas, turnips, etc.)	1 cup to 1½ cups	1 cup
Potatoes (white, sweet, yams)	1 medium to large (can fit in the palm of your hand)	1 medium (can fit in the palm of your hand)
Bread	2 slices	1 slice
English muffin	1–2 muffins	1 muffin
Berries	1–2 cups	1 cup
Grapefruit	½ to 1 grapefruit	½ grapefruit
Dried fruit	¼ cup	2 tablespoons

Slow Fuels

Here the measurement is a no-brainer. In fact, there is no measurement! Eat liberally from this food category, since slow fuels contain very few calories but lots of fiber and nutrition. Slow fuels will fill you up, too.

Fat Fuels

Your fat intake is taken care of primarily from the meats, eggs, oils, nuts, and seeds you eat. You do need to keep tabs on how much fat you eat, however, since it packs a lot of calories in a tiny food package. A serving of any of these fats is about the size of your thumb (that would be roughly a tablespoon). A teaspoon, roughly, would be the size of your fingertip.

CONTROL YOUR BODY COMPOSITION

Nutritionally, you can control your muscle development and overall fitness largely by the types of carbs you eat, either fast fuel or slow fuel. To get leaner, for example, you'd consume mostly slow-fuel sources as your primary carbohydrates. This happens in Block 1.

If you're very active—you work out intensely most days of the week—and you want to build a strong, athletic physique, you'd ramp up your consumption of fast fuels. These carbs provide you with more calories and insulin to rebuild muscle after hard workouts. On Block 3, you eat more fast-fuel carbs than you do on the other two blocks.

Remember, the Body Fuel plan shifts carb intake—and therefore calorie intake—from high to low, then back again, for a faster metabolism. Start the plan by following the three blocks as prescribed:

- Block 3: weeks 1–3
- Block 2: weeks 4–5
- Block 1: week 6

Once you have a firm understanding of how your body responds to the different blocks, feel free to make adjustments. That's what I mean by being your own nutritionist. Listen to your body, and tweak accordingly. Let me give you some scenarios of how to do this as you go along, based on your goals:

> *Scenario A.* You want to focus on gaining size or simply training hard. Stay on Block 3, with its higher fast-fuel carb intake, until you achieve the desired results. This might mean staying on Block 3 longer than three weeks. That's okay. In fact, I encourage it.

Scenario B. You've gained sufficient muscle, but you want to achieve more muscle definition. Taper down by switching to Block 2 for a while. For faster results, follow Block 1 after you've been on Block 2.

Scenario C. Your number one goal is weight loss, or maybe you exercise only a couple of times a week and are burning minimal calories. Your best bet is to switch between Block 2 and Block 1.

Scenario D. Although rare on this plan, a plateau might occur before you've reached your weight loss goal. A plateau is a stalemate in which you don't seem to be dropping pounds. If this happens, go on Block 1 for a week, ramp up your training, and see how your body responds.

Scenario E. You're close to your weight goal. It's only five or six pounds away. Switch to Block 1, and you'll get there in no time.

Scenario F. You've reached your goal weight. Now what? Block 3 is a good maintenance plan for most people, and you can add in some occasional treats such as desserts. You'll be able to eat those foods because they will get burned up by your supercharged metabolism and fuel-efficient body. But then again, you've got to listen to and watch your body. If your clothes are feeling tight again or if your weight is climbing, you need to get back on Block 2 or 1 and stay strict. Some people will need to use Block 2 as a maintenance plan. Give yourself a limit of five pounds over your goal weight that you will not exceed. If you do, get back on the program to keep your weight in check.

So you see, the Body Fuel plan is infinitely flexible. It works with your body to fuel your muscles and give you the shape and contour you want.

GROCERY SHOPPING FOR BODY FUEL

Body Fuel nutrition starts in the grocery store, so make a weekly date with your supermarket. Your mission: seek and purchase quality food to go along with each week of the Body Fuel plan. What you may or may not realize, however, is that the foods you buy have a direct influence on the quality of your workouts, the muscles you're trying to build, and the fat you're trying to burn.

Because the fittest shoppers are those armed with the most facts, I've compiled six weeks of shopping lists for you, based on the sample meal plans (see page 85). They give you an idea of what kinds of foods you shouldn't leave the store without. These lists are guidelines only; they may vary according to what you already have available in your fridge, freezer, or pantry. Feel free to modify the lists as you see fit.

THE BODY FUEL MEAL PLANS

Here are the sample meal plans for Block 3, Block 2, and Block 1. They include easy-to-prepare recipes, which are found in the next chapter. I've also included a meal plan template in the Appendix that you can use to create your own Body Fuel menus.

WEEKS 1–3: BLOCK 3

WEEK 1 • DAY 1

Breakfast (Fast Fuel)

2 slices Canadian bacon, pan-fried

1¼ cups packaged cereal such as Special K or a high-fiber cereal like raisin bran or Fiber One

1 cup almond milk for the cereal

Lunch (Fast Fuel)

Grilled Chicken and Vegetable Sandwich

Dinner (Fast Fuel)

Roast beef, such as eye of round (6–8 ounces for men, 3–5 ounces for women)

Asparagus sautéed in 1 tablespoon olive oil

1 baked potato, topped with 1–2 tablespoons nonfat sour cream, if desired

Snack 1 (Fast Fuel)

Egg Salad on Toast

Snack 2

Hard-boiled eggs (3–4 for men, 1–2 for women)

Handful of almonds

WEEK 1 • DAY 2

Breakfast (Fast Fuel)

Soft-boiled eggs (3–4 for men, 1–2 for women)

Oatmeal with Berries

Lunch (Fast Fuel)

Grilled chicken breast (6–8 ounces for men, 3–5 ounces for women), or leftover roast beef from the previous night's dinner

Brown rice, cooked (1 cup for men, ½ cup for women)

Tossed salad with 1–2 tablespoons low-fat salad dressing

Dinner (Fast Fuel)

Grilled or baked salmon (6–8 ounces for men, 3–5 ounces for women)

Kale sautéed in 1 tablespoon olive oil

1 baked sweet potato

Snack 1

½ grilled chicken breast

8 ounces *Fuelin' Veggie Juice*

Snack 2 (Fast Fuel)

Bananafana Cocoa Smoothie

WEEK 1 • DAY 3

Breakfast (Fast Fuel)

Scrambled Eggs with Tomatoes and Potatoes

Lunch (Fast Fuel)

Sautéed Shrimp and Citrus Salad

Dinner (Fast Fuel)

Pork Chop and Baby Broccoli

Couscous (1 cup for men, ½ cup for women)

Snack 1

½ chicken breast

Raw cut-up slow-fuel veggies

Snack 2 (Fast Fuel)

Carrot Cake Protein Bites

WEEK 1 • DAY 4

Breakfast (Fast Fuel)

Scrambled eggs (3–4 for men, 2 for women)

1 Roma tomato, sliced

Whole-grain or sprouted-grain toast (2 slices for men, 1 slice for women), with all-fruit jam, if desired

Lunch (Fast Fuel)

Ahi Tuna Salad

1 apple

Dinner (Fast Fuel)

Giant scallops (6–8 ounces for men, 3–5 ounces for women) sautéed in 1 tablespoon olive oil

1 cup stewed tomatoes

Brown rice, cooked (1 cup for men, ½ cup for women)

Snack 1

Hard-boiled eggs (3–4 for men, 1–2 for women)

Handful of almonds

Snack 2 (Fast Fuel)

Island Breeze Smoothie

WEEK 1 • DAY 5

Breakfast (Fast Fuel)

Mango Tango Smoothie

Lunch (Fast Fuel)

Caesar salad with sliced grilled or baked chicken breast (6–8 ounces for men, 3–5 ounces for women), romaine lettuce, and green bell pepper strips with 1–2 tablespoons low-fat Caesar salad dressing

1 peach or other seasonal fruit

Dinner (Fast Fuel)

Chicken Fajitas

Snack 1

Crab Salad on Avocado

Snack 2 (Fast Fuel)

Carrot Cake Protein Bites

WEEK 1 • DAY 6

Breakfast (Fast Fuel)

Open-Faced Egg Benedict

Lunch (Fast Fuel)

Lean ground beef patty (6–8 ounces for men, 3–5 ounces for women)

Tossed salad with 1–2 tablespoons low-fat salad dressing

Black beans, cooked (1 cup for men, ½ cup for women)

Dinner (Fast Fuel)

2 broiled veal chops (6–8 ounces for men, 3–5 ounces for women), topped with no-sugar-added pasta sauce

Zucchini sautéed in 1 tablespoon olive oil

Whole-wheat pasta, cooked (1 cup for men, ½ cup for women)

Snack 1

Asparagus Wrapped with Deli Turkey

Snack 2 (Fast Fuel)

Mango Tango Smoothie

WEEK 1 • DAY 7

Breakfast (Fast Fuel)

Scrambled eggs (3–4 for men, 2 for women)

1 Roma tomato, sliced

Grits, cooked (1 cup for men, ½ cup for women)

Lunch (Fast Fuel)

Breaded Chicken with Green Beans

Dinner (Fast Fuel)

Grilled Catfish with Coleslaw and Rice

Snack 1

2–3 ounces tuna

1 cup kale chips

Snack 2 (Fast Fuel)

Egg Salad on Toast

WEEK 1 SHOPPING LIST

Vegetables

Asparagus
Potatoes
Sweet potatoes
Onions
Garlic
Lettuce, such as iceberg or buttercrunch
Romaine lettuce
Fresh kale
Fresh spinach
Roma tomatoes
Tomatoes, such as beefsteak
Celery
Cucumber
Broccoli
Cauliflower
Zucchini
Cabbage
Green beans
Bell peppers: green, red, and yellow
Eggplant
Portobello mushroom
Jalapeños
Small bunch of cilantro
Carrots

Fruits

Pitted Medjool dates
Shredded coconut
Fresh berries: strawberries and blueberries
Apples
Peaches
Avocados
Bananas
Mango
Lime juice
Limes

Meat and Poultry

Canadian bacon
Beef roast (such as eye round)
Pork chops
Chicken breasts
Lean ground beef
Veal chops
Deli turkey

Seafood

Fillet of salmon
Shrimp
Giant scallops
Catfish

Eggs and Meat Alternatives

Eggs

Cereals, Grains, and Breads

Cereal such as Fiber One or Special K
Whole-grain bread
Oatmeal
Brown rice
Whole-wheat pasta
Grits
English muffins
French baguette
Flour tortillas

Frozen Foods

Frozen peaches
Frozen pineapple
Frozen mangoes

Canned Goods

Stewed tomatoes
Crabmeat
Black beans
Tuna

Oils and Vinegar

Low-fat or reduced-calorie salad dressing
Low-fat Caesar salad dressing
Olive oil
Apple cider vinegar
Rice vinegar
Mayonnaise

Spices

Salt
Ground cinnamon
Ground nutmeg
Ground cloves
Black pepper
Garlic powder

Onion powder
Chili powder
Cumin
Paprika
Cayenne
Vanilla extract

Condiments and Sweetening Agents

No-sugar-added pasta or marinara sauce
Raw organic agave nectar
Raw organic honey
Sugar
Mustard

Beverages

Almond milk, unsweetened
Chocolate almond milk

Miscellaneous

Raw almonds
Walnuts
Unsweetened applesauce
All-fruit jam
Kale chips
Plant-based chocolate protein powder
Plant-based vanilla protein powder
Chia seeds
Almond butter
Flaxseeds
Knorr Hollandaise sauce mix
Bread crumbs
Sesame seeds

WEEK 2 • DAY 8

Breakfast (Fast Fuel)

Open-Faced Breakfast Sandwich

Lunch (Fast Fuel)

Grilled Chicken and Vegetable Sandwich

Dinner (Fast Fuel)

2 grilled or broiled pork chops (6–8 ounces for men, 3–5 ounces for women) with teriyaki sauce
Steamed spinach
1 sweet potato, baked

Snack 1

Cucumber Cups

Snack 2 (Fast Fuel)

Very Berry Smoothie

WEEK 2 • DAY 9

Breakfast (Fast Fuel)

Goat Cheese Omelet

Whole-grain or sprouted-grain toast (2 slices for men, 1 slice for women), with all-fruit jam, if desired

Lunch (Fast Fuel)

Deli Turkey Pita Sandwich

Dinner (Fast Fuel)

Dinner out: sushi

Seaweed salad

Snack 1

½ grilled chicken breast

8 ounces *Fuelin' Veggie Juice*

Snack 2 (Fast Fuel)

Island Breeze Smoothie

WEEK 2 • DAY 10

Breakfast (Fast Fuel)

Mango Tango Smoothie

Lunch (Fast Fuel)

Salmon Barley Salad

Dinner (Fast Fuel)

Lean ground beef (6–8 ounces for men, 3–5 ounces for women), cooked in no-sugar-added marinara sauce and served over sautéed zucchini strips and whole-wheat pasta (1 cup for men, ½ cup for women)

Snack 1

½ chicken breast

Raw cut-up slow-fuel veggies

Snack 2 (Fast Fuel)

Sliced cucumbers dipped in hummus (1 cup for men, ½ cup for women)

WEEK 2 • DAY 11

Breakfast (Fast Fuel)

Zucchini Frittata

Lunch (Fast Fuel)

Sliced deli roast beef (6–8 ounces for men, 3–5 ounces for women) with 1 tablespoon mustard on rye bread (2 slices for men, 1 slice for women)

Dill pickle

Sliced tomato

Dinner (Fast Fuel)

Rotisserie chicken, skin removed (6–8 ounces for men, 3–5 ounces for women)

Shredded fresh cabbage dressed with 1 tablespoon low-fat mayonnaise and 2 tablespoons freshly squeezed lemon juice

Brown rice (1 cup for men, ½ cup for women)

Snack 1 (Fast Fuel)

Mango Tango Smoothie

Snack 2

Crab Salad on Avocado

WEEK 2 • DAY 12

Breakfast (Fast Fuel)

Hard-boiled eggs (3–4 for men, 2 for women)

Oatmeal with Berries

Lunch (Fast Fuel)

Leftover rotisserie chicken (6–8 ounces for men, 3–5 ounces for women)

Raw broccoli and cauliflower florets

Leftover brown rice (1 cup for men, ½ cup for women)

Dinner

2 grilled or broiled lamb chops (6–8 ounces for men, 3–5 ounces for women)

Roasted red bell peppers

Snack 1 (Fast Fuel)

Very Berry Smoothie

Snack 2 (Fast Fuel)

1 hard-boiled egg

1 medium apple

WEEK 2 • DAY 13

Breakfast (Fast Fuel)

Canadian bacon (4 slices for men, 2 slices for women), pan-fried

1¼ cups packaged cereal such as Special K or a high-fiber cereal like raisin bran or Fiber One

1 cup almond milk for the cereal

Lunch (Fast Fuel)

Tofu Singapore Noodles

Dinner (Fast Fuel)

Baked tilapia seasoned with lemon pepper

Roasted Brussels sprouts (spray with olive oil cooking spray and sprinkle with garlic salt prior to roasting)

Brown rice, cooked (1 cup for men, ½ cup for women)

Snack 1

Asparagus Wrapped with Deli Turkey

Snack 2 (Fast Fuel)

Mango Tango Smoothie

WEEK 2 • DAY 14

Breakfast (Fast Fuel)

Sunny-Side-Up Egg with Potatoes

Lunch (Fast Fuel)

Breaded Chicken with Green Beans (or leftover *Tofu Singapore Noodles*)

Dinner (Fast Fuel)

Sirloin steak (6–8 ounces for men, 3–5 ounces for women)

Tossed salad with 1–2 tablespoons low-fat salad dressing

1 baked potato, with 1–2 tablespoons sour cream, if desired

Snack 1

2–3 ounces tuna

1 cup kale chips

Snack 2 (Fast Fuel)

Island Breeze Smoothie

WEEK 2 SHOPPING LIST

Vegetables

Fresh spinach
Fresh kale
Sweet potatoes
Cucumbers
Zucchini
Assorted vegetables to eat raw: baby carrots, cauliflower, broccoli, cucumbers
Potatoes
Lettuce, such as iceberg or buttercrunch
Brussels sprouts
Asparagus
Tomatoes
Jalapeños
Mushrooms
Bell peppers: green and red
Eggplant
Green beans
Onion
Green onions
Bean sprouts
Flat-leaf parsley

Fruits

Apples
Bananas (unless you froze a couple from last week's shopping trip)
Strawberries and blueberries
Oranges
Cantaloupe
Mangoes
Avocados
Lemon juice

Meat and Poultry

Chicken breasts
Rotisserie chicken (pick up on day 11)
Lean ground beef
Lamb chops
Deli turkey meat
Deli ham
Sirloin steak

Seafood

Tilapia
Fillet of salmon

Eggs and Meat Alternatives

Eggs
Tofu

Cereals, Grains, and Breads

Barley
Rye bread
Couscous
French baguette
Rice vermicelli
Pita bread

Frozen Foods

Frozen blueberries, unsweetened

Canned Goods

Crabmeat
Tuna

Oils and Vinegar

Low-fat mayonnaise
Olive oil cooking spray

Spices

Lemon pepper
Garlic salt
Curry powder

Condiments

Teriyaki sauce
Soy sauce
Cholula sauce
Dijon mustard

Miscellaneous

Goat cheese
Grated cheddar cheese
Hummus
Dill pickles
Sour cream
Pumpkin seeds
Seitan

WEEK 3 • DAY 15

Breakfast (Fast Fuel)

Soft-boiled eggs (3–4 for men, 2 for women)

Oatmeal with Berries

Lunch (Fast Fuel)

Grilled chicken (6–8 ounces for men, 3–5 ounces for women)

Tossed salad of romaine lettuce, cherry tomatoes, chopped celery, and other salad vegetables with 1–2 tablespoons low-fat salad dressing

Brown rice, cooked (1 cup for men, ½ cup for women)

Dinner (Fast Fuel)

Seafood Mango Salad

Snack 1

Crab Salad on Avocado

Snack 2 (Fast Fuel)

Very Berry Smoothie

WEEK 3 • DAY 16

Breakfast (Fast Fuel)

Turkey sausage links or patties (4 for men, 2 for women), pan-fried

Whole-grain or sprouted-grain toast (2 slices for men, 1 slice for women), spread with all-fruit jam, if desired

Lunch (Fast Fuel)

Broccoli Salad, or leftover grilled chicken and a slow-fuel vegetable such as a sliced tomato

Brown rice, cooked (1 cup for men, ½ cup for women)

Dinner (Fast Fuel)

Hearty Steak and Potatoes

Tossed salad with 1–2 tablespoons low-fat salad dressing

Snack 1

1 hard-boiled egg

Handful of almonds

Snack 2 (Fast Fuel)

Very Berry Smoothie

WEEK 3 • DAY 17

Breakfast (Fast Fuel)

Zucchini Frittata

Lunch

Tuna, canned (6–8 ounces for men, 3–5 ounces for women)

Buttercrunch lettuce and other salad veggies, plus chickpeas (1 cup for men, ½ cup for women)

1–2 tablespoons low-fat salad dressing

Dinner (Fast Fuel)

Pork Chop with Baby Broccoli

1 baked sweet potato

Snack 1 (Fast Fuel)

Egg Salad on Toast

Snack 2 (Fast Fuel)

1 slice deli turkey

1 medium apple

WEEK 3 • DAY 18

Breakfast (Fast Fuel)

Open-Faced Egg Benedict

Lunch (Fast Fuel)

Salad bar: 1–2 cups fresh greens, ½ cup chopped ham, kidney beans or chickpeas (1 cup for men, ½ cup for women), tomato slices, chopped green bell pepper, 1 tablespoon sunflower seeds, 1–2 tablespoons low-fat salad dressing

Dinner (Fast Fuel)

Chicken Fajitas

Snack 1

Asparagus Wrapped with Deli Turkey

Snack 2 (Fast Fuel)

Mango Tango Smoothie

WEEK 3 • DAY 19

Breakfast (Fast Fuel)

Canadian bacon (4 slices for men, 2 slices for women), pan-fried

Oatmeal, cooked (1 cup for men, ½ cup for women)

Lunch (Fast Fuel)

Roasted or deli turkey (6–8 ounces for men, 3–5 ounces for women) with 1 tablespoon mustard on rye bread (2 slices for men, 1 slice for women)

1 dill pickle

1–2 cups raw broccoli or cauliflower

Dinner (Fast Fuel)

Sausage-Stuffed Zucchini with Orzo

Snack 1

2–3 ounces leftover turkey

Raw cut-up slow-fuel veggies

Snack 2 (Fast Fuel)

Bananafana Cocoa Smoothie

WEEK 3 • DAY 20

Breakfast (Fast Fuel)

Scrambled Eggs with Tomatoes and Potatoes

Lunch (Fast Fuel)

Salmon, canned (6–8 ounces for men, 3–5 ounces for women)

2 cups salad greens with 1–2 tablespoons low-fat salad dressing

Whole-grain or sprouted-grain bread (2 slices for men, 1 slice for women)

Dinner (Fast Fuel)

Asian takeout of mixed steamed vegetables and shrimp (2 cups for men, 1 cup for women)

Brown rice, cooked (1 cup for men, ½ cup for women)

Snack 1

Asparagus Wrapped with Deli Turkey

Snack 2 (Fast Fuel)

Island Breeze Smoothie

WEEK 3 • DAY 21

Breakfast (Fast Fuel)

Bananafana Cocoa Smoothie

Lunch (Fast Fuel)

Lean ground beef patty (6–8 ounces for men, 3–5 ounces for women), pan-fried, or leftover Asian takeout

1 cup stewed tomatoes

1 baked potato

Dinner (Fast Fuel)

2 broiled lamb chops (6–8 ounces for men, 3–5 ounces for women)

Tossed salad with 1–2 tablespoons low-fat salad dressing

Couscous, cooked (1 cup for men, ½ cup for women)

Snack 1

Crab Salad on Avocado

Snack 2 (Fast Fuel)

Egg Salad on Toast

WEEK 3 SHOPPING LIST

Vegetables

Lettuce, such as iceberg or buttercrunch

Romaine lettuce

Celery

Broccoli

Potatoes

Sweet potatoes

Zucchini

Asparagus

Cauliflower

Assorted vegetables to eat raw: baby carrots and cucumbers

Tomatoes, such as beefsteak

Roma tomatoes

Cherry tomatoes

Broccoli

Bell peppers: green, red, and yellow

Jalapeños

Serrano chile

Radishes

Jicama

Flat-leaf parsley

Fruits

Berries: strawberries and blueberries (unless you froze leftover berries from the previous week)

Mango

Avocados

Bananas

Limes

Meat and Poultry

Chicken breasts

Turkey sausage

Pork chops

Steak

Canadian bacon

Italian sausage links

Lean ground beef

Lamb chops

Deli ham

Deli turkey

Sirloin steak

Seafood

Squid

Shrimp

Eggs and Meat Alternatives

Eggs

Cereals, Grains, and Breads

Whole-grain or sprouted-grain bread

Orzo

Small flour tortillas

Canned Goods

Crabmeat

Tuna

Salmon

Chickpeas

Stewed tomatoes

Oils and Vinegar

Red wine vinegar

Miscellaneous

Kale chips

Parmesan cheese

Hoo-ya!

Love Those Leftovers

Most of us are on tight budgets. Often, the idea of fixing tasty, healthful meals on a regular basis can seem daunting. But it's doable—and immensely cheaper than eating out all the time.

With some foresight and organization, you can enjoy the proverbial champagne lifestyle while cooking on a beer budget. To start, here are some basic ideas for economical but healthy eating:

Freeze fruits. Sometimes bananas get so ripe, you want to throw them out. I like to peel them, wrap them up, and stash them in the freezer. Frozen bananas make great smoothies. Another fruit that freezes well are grapes. Take them out when you want a cold, fruity treat. Freezing also works well for berries (raspberries, blueberries, pitted cherries, and so forth), which tend to go bad in a relatively short amount of time if you keep them in the fridge.

Freeze leftovers. Did you fix a meal so big that you've got leftover food? Package those leftovers in individual servings and freeze them right away. Whenever you cook, figure out how to double the recipe, then freeze the extras in meal-sized portions to save time and money.

Leftovers as lunch or snacks. Last night's dinner makes today's great lunch. Some of my favorite lunches are good leftovers. Maybe add new things to spice it up, such as fresh vegetables or a side of fruit. If a small portion of leftovers isn't enough for a meal, it might make a good snack.

Brown-bag it. This saves money and gives you lots of healthful lunch options. A whole-wheat pita pocket filled with veggies or last night's leftovers and fruit are good brown-bag choices.

Boil up some eggs. Hard-boil eggs so you'll have a batch on hand. They're good on bread and on salads.

Save food. Old vegetables can be added to stews or stocks. Tomatoes can be pureed into tomato sauce or salsa.

Soup's on. Look to serve your family soup once a week. Soup is the ultimate money stretcher. Using the aforementioned preplanned menu, you can simmer the roasted chicken carcass from Monday's meal for stock, add leftover vegetables, beans, or lentils, and serve with salad and bread for a tasty meal that can save $10–$12 each week.

WEEKS 4–5: BLOCK 2

WEEK 4 • DAY 1

Breakfast (Fast Fuel)

Canadian bacon (4 slices for men, 2 slices for women), pan-fried

1¼ cups packaged cereal such as Special K or a high-fiber cereal like raisin bran or Fiber One

1 cup almond milk for the cereal

Lunch (Fast Fuel)

Grilled Chicken and Vegetable Sandwich

Dinner

Grilled sirloin steak

Mashed Cauliflower

Snack 1

Celery with almond butter

Snack 2

Hard-boiled egg

Handful of almonds

WEEK 4 • DAY 2

Breakfast (Fast Fuel)

Soft-boiled eggs (4 for men, 2 for women)

Oatmeal with Berries

Lunch (Fast Fuel)

Deli Turkey Pita Sandwich

Dinner

Grilled or baked salmon (6–8 ounces for men, 3–5 ounces for women)

Kale sautéed in 1 tablespoon olive oil

Yellow wax beans

Snack 1

1 hard-boiled egg

Handful of almonds

Snack 2

½ grilled chicken breast

8 ounces *Fuelin' Veggie Juice*

WEEK 4 • DAY 3

Breakfast (Fast Fuel)

Turkey sausage patties or links (4 pieces for men, 2 pieces for women), pan-fried

Whole-grain or sprouted-grain toast (2 slices for men, 1 slice for women), with all-fruit jam, if desired

Lunch (Fast Fuel)

Ahi Tuna Salad

1 medium apple

Dinner

Pork Chop with Baby Broccoli

Snack 1

Cucumber Cups (stuff with tuna or chicken)

Snack 2

Crab Salad on Avocado

WEEK 4 • DAY 4

Breakfast (Fast Fuel)

Scrambled eggs (4 for men, 2 for women)

1 Roma tomato, sliced

¼ of a cantaloupe

Lunch (Fast Fuel)

Sautéed Shrimp and Citrus Salad

Dinner

Giant scallops (6–8 ounces for men, 3–5 ounces for women), sautéed in 1 tablespoon olive oil

1 cup stewed tomatoes

Tossed salad with 1–2 tablespoons low-fat salad dressing

Snack 1

Cucumber Cups (stuff with tuna or chicken)

Snack 2

Asparagus Wrapped with Deli Turkey

WEEK 4 • DAY 5

Breakfast (Fast Fuel)

Bananafana Cocoa Smoothie

Lunch (Fast Fuel)

Tofu Singapore Noodles

Dinner

Grilled Flank Steak with Grilled Vegetable Salad

Snack 1

1 hard-boiled egg

Handful of almonds

Snack 2

2–3 ounces tuna or leftover flank steak

1 cup kale chips

WEEK 4 • DAY 6

Breakfast (Fast Fuel)

Baked Egg with Mushrooms

Whole-grain or sprouted-grain toast (2 slices for men, 1 slice for women), with all-fruit jam, if desired

Lunch (Fast Fuel)

Cooked lean ground beef, cooked kidney beans (1 cup for men, ½ cup for women), and tomato sauce and spices, mixed together to make a quick chili

Dinner

Seafood restaurant dinner, with grilled salmon or other fish

Steamed side vegetables

Tossed salad with oil and vinegar dressing

Snack 1

½ chicken breast

1 cup kale chips

Snack 2

1 hard-boiled egg

Handful of almonds

WEEK 4 • DAY 7

Breakfast (Fast Fuel)

Scrambled eggs (4 for men, 2 for women)

1 Roma tomato, sliced

Cooked grits (1 cup for men, ½ cup for women)

Lunch (Fast Fuel)

Broccoli Salad or leftover salmon from last night's restaurant dinner

1 baked sweet potato

Dinner

Roast turkey breast (6–8 ounces for men, 3–5 ounces for women)

Mashed Cauliflower

Tossed salad with 1–2 tablespoons low-fat salad dressing

Snack 1

2–3 ounces leftover turkey breast

8 ounces *Fuelin' Veggie Juice*

Snack 2

1 hard-boiled egg

Handful of almonds

WEEK 4 SHOPPING LIST

Vegetables

Celery
Cauliflower
Fresh kale
Fresh spinach
Lettuce
Mixed salad greens
Broccoli
Roma tomatoes
Cherry tomatoes
Asparagus
Sweet potatoes
Onions
Red onions
Mushrooms
Portobello mushrooms
Eggplant
Bell peppers: red and green
Zucchini
Cucumbers
Bean sprouts
Carrots
Fresh mint
Fresh rosemary

Fruits

Strawberries and blueberries
Bananas
Apples, such as Gala
Avocados
Cantaloupe
Grapefruit
Oranges

Meat and Poultry

Chicken breasts
Sirloin steak
Deli turkey
Turkey sausage
Pork chops
Flank steak
Lean ground beef
Turkey breast

Seafood

Salmon fillet
Giant scallops
Shrimp
Tuna steak

Eggs and Meat Alternatives

Eggs
Tofu

Cereals, Grains, and Breads

Pita bread
French baguette

Frozen Foods

Yellow wax beans

Canned Goods

Crabmeat
Kidney beans
Tomato sauce
Stewed tomatoes

Oils and Vinegar

Butter

Spices

Chili powder
Cayenne

Beverages

Almond milk, unsweetened
Milk

Miscellaneous

Almond butter
Raw almonds

WEEK 5 • DAY 8

Breakfast (Fast Fuel)

Eggs with Green Beans and Ham

Cooked grits (1 cup for men, ½ cup for women)

Lunch (Fast Fuel)

Grilled Chicken and Vegetable Sandwich

Dinner

2 grilled or broiled pork chops (6–8 ounces for men, 3–5 ounces for women) with teriyaki sauce

Steamed yellow squash

Steamed spinach

Snack 1

½ chicken breast

Raw cut-up slow-fuel veggies

Snack 2

1 hard-boiled egg

Handful of almonds

WEEK 5 • DAY 9

Breakfast

Goat Cheese Omelet

Lunch (Fast Fuel)

Grilled Chicken and Spinach

Cooked brown rice (1 cup for men, ½ cup for women)

Dinner

Asian takeout of mixed steamed vegetables and shrimp (2 cups for men, 1 cup for women)

Snack 1 (Fast Fuel)

Island Breeze Smoothie

Snack 2

Crab Salad on Avocado

WEEK 5 • DAY 10

Breakfast (Fast Fuel)

Open-Faced Breakfast Sandwich

Lunch

Club Salad

Dinner

Lean ground beef (6–8 ounces for men, 3–5 ounces for women), cooked in no-sugar-added marinara sauce and served over sautéed zucchini

Snack 1 (Fast Fuel)

Tango Mango Smoothie

Snack 2

Cucumber Cups (stuff with tuna or chicken)

WEEK 5 • DAY 11

Breakfast (Fast Fuel)

Zucchini Frittata

½ grapefruit

Lunch (Fast Fuel)

Sliced deli roast beef (6–8 ounces for men, 3–5 ounces for women) with 1 tablespoon mustard on rye bread (2 slices for men, 1 slice for women)

Dill pickle

Sliced tomato

Dinner

Rotisserie chicken, skin removed (6–8 ounces for men, 3–5 ounces for women)

Shredded fresh cabbage dressed with 1 tablespoon low-fat mayonnaise and 2 tablespoons freshly squeezed lemon juice

Snack 1

Asparagus Wrapped with Deli Turkey

Snack 2

1 hard-boiled egg

Handful of almonds

WEEK 5 • DAY 12

Breakfast (Fast Fuel)

Sunny-Side-Up Egg with Potatoes

Lunch (Fast Fuel)

Leftover rotisserie chicken (6–8 ounces for men, 3–5 ounces for women)

Raw broccoli and cauliflower florets

1 medium apple

Dinner

Grilled or broiled lamb chops (6–8 ounces for men, 3–5 ounces for women)

Roasted red bell peppers

Cucumber salad: ½ cucumber, chopped, dressed with 1 tablespoon olive oil and 2 tablespoons raspberry vinegar

Snack 1

2–3 ounces tuna

1 cup kale chips

Snack 2

Celery with almond butter

WEEK 5 • DAY 13

Breakfast (Fast Fuel)

Open-Faced Breakfast Sandwich

Lunch (Fast Fuel)

Breaded Chicken with Green Beans

Dinner

Baked tilapia (6–8 ounces for men, 3–5 ounces for women), seasoned with lemon pepper

Roasted Brussels sprouts (spray with olive oil cooking spray and sprinkle with garlic salt prior to roasting)

Tossed salad with 1–2 tablespoons low-fat salad dressing

Snack 1 (Fast Fuel)

Bananafana Cocoa Smoothie

Snack 2

½ grilled chicken breast or 2–3 ounces leftover tilapia

8 ounces *Fuelin' Veggie Juice*

WEEK 5 • DAY 14

Breakfast (Fast Fuel)

Scrambled Eggs with Tomatoes and Potatoes

Lunch (Fast Fuel)

Grilled Chicken and Vegetable Sandwich

Dinner

Grilled sirloin steak

Mashed Cauliflower

Tossed salad with 1–2 tablespoons low-fat salad dressing

Snack 1

1 hard-boiled egg

Handful of almonds

Snack 2

½ chicken breast

Assorted raw cut-up slow-fuel veggies

WEEK 5 SHOPPING LIST

Vegetables

Green beans
Fresh spinach
Yellow squash
Assorted vegetables to eat raw: baby carrots, cauliflower, broccoli, cucumbers
Zucchini
Yellow squash
Celery
Tomatoes, such as beefsteak
Cherry tomatoes
Bell peppers: red and green
Mushrooms
Portobello mushrooms
Eggplant
Onions
Carrots
Lettuce, such as iceberg or buttercrunch
Romaine lettuce
Brussels sprouts
Potatoes
Cauliflower
Garlic
Asparagus
Cucumbers

Fruits

Avocados
Mangoes
Apples
Cantaloupe

Meat and Poultry

Ham
Chicken breasts
Pork chops
Lean ground beef
Deli roast beef
Rotisserie chicken
Lamb chops
Sirloin steak
Bacon

Seafood

Tilapia

Eggs and Meat Alternatives

Eggs

Cereals, Grains, and Breads

French baguette

Canned Goods

Crabmeat
Tuna

Oils and Vinegar

Balsamic vinegar
Raspberry vinegar

Miscellaneous

Hummus
Goat cheese

WEEK 6: BLOCK 1

WEEK 6 • DAY 1

Breakfast

Goat Cheese Omelet

Lunch

Chicken Vegetable Soup

Dinner

Grilled Flank Steak and Grilled Vegetable Salad

Snack 1

Crab Salad on Avocado

Snack 2 (Fast Fuel)

Bananafana Cocoa Smoothie

WEEK 6 • DAY 2

Breakfast (Fast Fuel)

Turkey sausage links or patties (4 pieces for men, 2 pieces for women), pan-fried

Whole-grain or sprouted-grain toast (2 slices for men, 1 slice for women), with all-fruit jam, if desired

Lunch

Broccoli Salad

Dinner

Grilled Herb Chicken with Brussels Sprouts

Snack 1

1 hard-boiled egg

Handful of almonds

Snack 2

½ grilled chicken breast

8 ounces *Fuelin' Veggie Juice*

WEEK 6 • DAY 3

Breakfast (Fast Fuel)

Bananafana Cocoa Smoothie

Lunch

Ahi Tuna Salad

Dinner

Chicken and Vegetable Skewers

Snack 1

1 hard-boiled egg

Handful of almonds

Snack 2

Cucumber Cups (stuff with tuna or chicken)

WEEK 6 • DAY 4

Breakfast

Goat Cheese Omelet

Lunch

Salad bar: 1–2 cups fresh greens, ½ cup kidney beans or chickpeas, tomato slices, chopped green pepper, 1 tablespoon sunflower seeds, 1–2 tablespoons low-fat salad dressing

Dinner

Naked Chicken Burrito

Snack 1

Asparagus Wrapped with Deli Turkey

Snack 2 (Fast Fuel)

Island Breeze Smoothie

WEEK 6 • DAY 5

Breakfast (Fast Fuel)

Canadian bacon (4 slices for men, 2 slices for women), pan-fried

Cooked oatmeal (1 cup for men, ½ cup for women)

Lunch

Roasted or deli turkey (6–8 ounces for men, 3–5 ounces for women)

1 dill pickle

1–2 cups raw broccoli or cauliflower florets

Dinner

Pork Chop with Baby Broccoli

Snack 1

2–3 ounces leftover turkey

Assorted raw cut-up slow-fuel veggies

Snack 2

1 hard-boiled egg

1 cup kale chips

WEEK 6 • DAY 6

Breakfast (Fast Fuel)

Zucchini Frittata

Lunch

Club Salad

Dinner

Asian takeout of mixed steamed vegetables and shrimp (2 cups for men, 1 cup for women)

Snack 1

Asparagus Wrapped with Deli Turkey

Snack 2

1 hard-boiled egg

Handful of almonds

WEEK 6 • DAY 7

Breakfast (Fast Fuel)

Mango Tango Smoothie

Lunch

Lean ground beef patty (6–8 ounces for men, 3–5 ounces for women)

1 cup stewed tomatoes

1 cup Italian green beans

Dinner

Broiled lamb chops (6–8 ounces for men, 3–5 ounces for women)

Mashed Cauliflower

Tossed salad with 1–2 tablespoons low-fat salad dressing

Snack 1

Crab Salad on Avocado

Snack 2

Zucchini Pancakes with Smoked Salmon

WEEK 6 SHOPPING LIST

Vegetables

Broccoli
Fresh spinach
Fresh kale
Mixed salad greens
Brussels sprouts
Cucumbers
Asparagus
Cauliflower
Assorted vegetables to eat raw: baby carrots, celery, and cherry or grape tomatoes
Zucchini
Tomatoes, any type
Green beans
Potato
Bell peppers: green and red
Mushrooms
Carrots
Red onion
Romaine lettuce
Jalapeños
Eggplant
Portobello mushrooms
Fresh rosemary
Fresh thyme
Flat-leaf parsley
Cilantro

Fruits

Avocados
Mangoes
Bananas
Cantaloupe
Lemons

Meat and Poultry

Chicken breasts
Flank steak
Turkey sausage
Canadian bacon
Deli turkey
Pork chops
Lean ground beef
Lamb chops

Seafood

Smoked salmon
Tuna steak

Eggs and Meat Alternatives

Eggs

Cereals, Grains, and Breads

Whole-grain or sprouted-grain bread

Canned Goods

Chicken broth	Stewed tomatoes	Black beans
Crabmeat	Italian green beans	

Spices

Poultry seasoning	Dried parsley	Crushed red pepper

Beverages

Almond milk, unsweetened

Miscellaneous

Goat cheese	Flour

If you're ready to try your hand at planning out your own meals, see my Body Fuel meal planning template in the Appendix. It's a helpful guide to make sure you get all the nutrition you need in every block.

CHAPTER 8

BODY FUEL RECIPES

I've been training as an athlete for over twenty-five years, and for over a decade I've trained elite Special Operations forces and many hundreds of thousands of men and women around the world. Naturally, as a leader in the fitness industry, I pay close and strict attention to what, how much, and when I eat. That's my job! Even so, I love to eat, and I love good food.

Since featuring recipes on my website (marklauren.com), and now on the pages of this book, I've been on the lookout for creative substitutions that will cut the amount of fat, calories, or salt without altering the flavor and consistency of the foods I love. I think I've succeeded, based on the positive comments from people on recipes I've dished up for them so far.

In creating recipes, I try to follow four rules: they've got to be easy to fix, intensely flavored, made with the freshest and best ingredients possible, and quick to prepare. And for anyone watching a food budget, I like to offer recipes that are affordable and won't break the household bank.

In my travels, one of the main gripes I hear from people trying to get in shape is that healthful eating can be bland and boring. Let me see a quick show of hands: who's craving a plain baked chicken breast right now? Exactly my point. No one.

Boring-as-hell diet food doesn't ring my bells, either. Let me assure you, too, that just because these recipes are in a diet book, they're not all about watery bits of lettuce and that ubiquitous fit-person staple, the unadorned chicken breast. I definitely couldn't live on that stuff, and you can't, either.

So forget all that nonsense. I've banished the boring factor and have come up with a series of recipes you'll love—and love to make. As a very useful addition, each of the recipes has its nutritional content listed, including calories per portion, in case you like to count those. My hope is to provide you with delicious and nutritious recipes that will satisfy your palate and keep you on the right track. All the recipes are so simple that you can whip them up even if you have no previous cooking experience.

Here's to healthful but never boring eating!

SMOOTHIES

Bananafana Cocoa Smoothie

MAKES 2 SERVINGS

2 scoops chocolate plant-based protein powder
2 medium bananas
2 tablespoons rolled oats
1 cup chocolate almond milk
1 tablespoon almond butter
1 teaspoon agave
1 tablespoon chia seeds
1 cup ice cubes
¼ teaspoon cinnamon (optional)

Place all ingredients in a blender. Add ½ cup water. Blend until smooth.

Nutrition: 276 calories per serving, 19 grams protein, 32 grams carbohydrate, and 8 grams fat.

Island Breeze Smoothie

MAKES 2 SERVINGS

2 scoops vanilla plant-based protein powder
1 cup almond milk
1 cup frozen peaches
½ medium banana
½ cup frozen pineapple
1 cup kale
1 handful spinach
1 tablespoon flaxseeds
1 tablespoon almond butter

Place all ingredients in a blender. Add ½ cup water. Blend until smooth.

Nutrition: 338 calories per serving, 28 grams protein, 34 grams carbohydrate, and 10 grams fat.

Mango Tango Smoothie

MAKES 2 SERVINGS

1 cup almond milk
1 cup frozen peaches
1 cup frozen mango
2 scoops vanilla plant-based protein powder
1 tablespoon almond butter

Place all ingredients in a blender. Add ½ cup water. Blend until smooth.

Nutrition: 332 calories per serving, 27 grams protein, 29 grams carbohydrate, and 12 grams fat.

Very Berry Smoothie

MAKES 2 SERVINGS

1 cup almond milk
1 cup frozen blueberries
½ cup ice
2 tablespoon old-fashioned oats
2 scoops vanilla plant-based protein powder
1 tablespoon chia seeds
2 teaspoons honey

Place all ingredients in a blender. Blend until smooth.

Nutrition: 299 calories per serving, 26 grams protein, 33 grams carbohydrate, and 7 grams fat.

HIGH-CALORIE SMOOTHIES

Banana Split Smoothie

MAKES 2 SERVINGS

1 cup strawberries
1 banana
2 scoops butter pecan ice cream
1 drop vanilla extract
2 scoops vanilla weight-gain powder
1 cup milk
2 scoops soy protein
1 tablespoon wheat germ
½ cup ice

Place all ingredients in a blender. Blend until smooth.

Nutrition: 525 calories per serving, 35 grams protein, 60 grams carbohydrate, and 15 grams fat.

Chocolate Almond Butter Smoothie

MAKES 2 SERVINGS

1 cup chocolate whole milk
2 scoops chocolate protein powder
1 tablespoon almond butter
1 tablespoon chia seeds
1 tablespoon flaxseeds
2 scoops butter pecan ice cream
½ cup ice

Place all ingredients in a blender. Blend until smooth.

Nutrition: 464 calories per serving, 31 grams protein, 40 grams carbohydrate, and 20 grams fat.

Oatmeal with Berries

MAKES 1 SERVING

½ cup oats
¼ cup blueberries
¼ cup strawberries
2 tablespoons honey
¼ teaspoon cinnamon
1 tablespoon chia seeds
1 tablespoon flaxseeds

In a pot, boil 1¼ cups water and stir in oats. Cook for 5 minutes over medium heat, stirring occasionally. Place oatmeal in a bowl and top with blueberries, strawberries, honey, cinnamon, chia seeds, and flaxseeds.

Nutrition: 422 calories per serving, 10 grams protein, 89 grams carbohydrate, and 9 grams fat.

Scrambled Eggs with Tomatoes and Potatoes

MAKES 1 SERVING

2 eggs
Salt
Black pepper
2 tablespoons olive oil
2 tablespoons chopped onion
1 clove garlic, minced
1 tomato, chopped
1 potato, diced

Beat eggs in a bowl until well blended. Season with salt and pepper.

Heat 1 tablespoon oil in nonstick skillet over medium heat. Add onion and garlic. Cook for 1 to 2 minutes.

Pour egg mixture into skillet with garlic and onion. Stir gently. Add tomato and cook until the mixture forms soft curds.

In another skillet, over medium heat, heat the remaining 1 tablespoon oil. Add diced potato. Cook for 10 to 13 minutes, until potato is brown and tender. Serve potato with scrambled eggs.

Nutrition: 332 calories per serving, 9.5 grams protein, 21.3 grams carbohydrate, and 23.2 grams fat.

Note: To increase calories, increase serving size to 1½ servings.

Open-Faced Egg Benedict

MAKES 1 SERVING

1 teaspoon vinegar
1 poached egg
½ toasted English muffin
1 slice Canadian bacon
1 slice tomato
3 slices avocado
1 tablespoon Hollandaise sauce, prepared from 1 package of Knorr Hollandaise sauce mix
1 teaspoon chopped flat-leaf parsley

To 1 inch of water in a pot, add the vinegar. Bring the water to a simmer. Crack egg in a bowl and pour it into the simmering water. Let the egg cook for 4 to 5 minutes. Remove the egg with a spatula.

Layer English muffin with Canadian bacon, tomato, avocado, and poached egg. Spoon Hollandaise sauce over poached egg. Sprinkle with parsley.

Nutrition: 272 calories per serving, 13.8 grams protein, 10.8 grams carbohydrate, and 11.4 grams fat.

Open-Faced Breakfast Sandwich

MAKES 1 SERVING

½ teaspoon olive oil
2 eggs
Salt
Black pepper
2 slices deli ham
1 slice whole-wheat bread
¼ cup baby spinach

Heat oil in a skillet over medium-high heat. Add eggs to skillet. Season with salt and pepper. Reduce heat to low and cook for 2 to 3 minutes, until egg whites and yolks are set. Remove eggs to a plate.

Heat deli ham in the skillet until hot, and toast the bread.

Place baby spinach over toast and top with ham. Place eggs on top.

Nutrition: 300 calories per serving, 28 grams protein, 5.3 grams carbohydrate, and 18.5 grams fat.

Note: To increase calories, increase serving size to 1½ servings.

Sunny-Side-Up Egg with Potatoes

MAKES 1 SERVING

1½ tablespoons olive oil
1 small potato, peeled and sliced
Salt
Black pepper
6 asparagus spears
1 egg
Cholula sauce
Orange wedges

Heat ½ tablespoon oil in skillet over medium-high heat. Add potato and cook for 5 to 6 minutes, or until brown and tender. Season with salt and pepper, then set aside.

Heat another ½ tablespoon oil in a skillet over medium-high heat. Add asparagus and season with salt and pepper. Cook for 3 to 4 minutes.

Heat the remaining ½ tablespoon oil in a skillet over medium-high heat. Add egg to the skillet. Sprinkle the egg with salt and pepper. Reduce heat to low and cook for 2 to 3 minutes, until egg white and yolk are set.

Place the potato and asparagus on a plate, and place the egg on top of the asparagus. Top egg with Cholula sauce. Serve with orange wedges.

Nutrition: 213 calories per serving, 7.3 grams protein, 18.8 grams carbohydrate, and 21.1 grams fat.

Zucchini Frittata

MAKES 1 SERVING

For the Salsa

1 tomato, chopped
1 teaspoon chopped jalapeño
1 teaspoon lime juice
1 tablespoon chopped cilantro

For the Frittata

½ tablespoon olive oil
½ cup peeled and sliced potato
⅓ cup chopped onion
¼ cup sliced zucchini
2 eggs
Salt
Black pepper
1 tablespoon cheddar cheese
2 slices cantaloupe

In a bowl, combine all the ingredients for the salsa. Set aside.

Preheat the oven to 400 degrees.

Heat the oil in a skillet over medium-high heat. Add potato and cook for 3 to 4 minutes. Transfer to a bowl.

To the same heated skillet, add the onion and zucchini. Cook for 2 minutes.

Beat the eggs in a bowl. Season with salt and pepper, then add the zucchini, onion, potato, and cheese.

Grease a ramekin with a little bit of olive oil and pour the egg mixture into the ramekin. Bake for 15 to 17 minutes.

Remove the frittata from the ramekin and transfer to a plate. Serve with salsa and cantaloupe.

Nutrition: 394 calories per serving, 18.5 grams protein, 34.8 grams carbohydrate, and 20.1 grams fat.

SLOW-FUEL BREAKFASTS

Eggs with Sautéed Zucchini and Yellow Squash

MAKES 1 SERVING

2 teaspoons olive oil
¼ cup sliced onion
½ cup sliced zucchini
½ cup sliced yellow squash
Salt
Black pepper
2 eggs

Heat 1 teaspoon oil in a skillet over medium heat. Add onion and cook for 1 to 2 minutes. Add zucchini and yellow squash and cook for 3 to 5 minutes, until vegetables are tender. Season with salt and pepper.

Heat the remaining 1 teaspoon oil in a skillet over medium heat. Reduce heat to low. Add eggs and cook for 2 to 3 minutes, until egg whites and yolks are set. Season with salt and pepper. Serve eggs with vegetables.

Nutrition: 268 calories per serving, 15 grams protein, 16 grams carbohydrate, and 16 grams fat.
Note: To increase calories, increase serving size to 1½ servings.

Eggs with Green Beans and Ham

MAKES 1 SERVING

Salt
1 cup green beans, cut into 1-inch lengths
2 eggs
Black pepper
½ tablespoon olive oil
¼ cup diced ham

Fill a small pot halfway with water. Bring to a boil and add salt and green beans. Cook for 5 to 6 minutes. Drain beans well.

Beat eggs in a bowl. Season with salt and pepper.

Heat oil in a skillet over medium heat. Add green beans and ham. Cook for 2 to 3 minutes. Pour in egg mixture, stir gently, and cook until egg mixture is no longer runny.

Nutrition: 272 calories, 26 grams protein, 15 grams carbohydrate, and 12 grams fat.

Note: To increase calories, increase serving size to 1½ servings.

Baked Egg with Mushrooms

MAKES 1 SERVING

½ tablespoon olive oil
¼ cup sliced onion
1 cup sliced mushrooms
Salt
Black pepper
1 egg

Preheat the oven to 400 degrees.

Heat oil in skillet over medium-high heat. Add onion and mushrooms. Cook for 2 to 3 minutes. Season with salt and pepper.

Place mushroom and onion mixture in a ramekin. Crack the egg on top. Bake for 10 to 12 minutes, until egg white is firm and egg yolk is soft. Season with additional salt and pepper.

Nutrition: 201 calories, 7.3 grams protein, 14.3 grams carbohydrate, and 12.8 grams fat.

Goat Cheese Omelet

MAKES 1 SERVING

1 tablespoon olive oil
2 tablespoons chopped onion
¼ cup sliced mushrooms
¼ cup chopped green bell pepper
¼ cup chopped red bell pepper
¼ cup spinach
1 egg
2 egg whites
Salt
Black pepper
1 tablespoon goat cheese

Heat ½ tablespoon oil in a skillet over medium-high heat. Add onion, mushrooms, bell peppers, and spinach and cook for 2 to 3 minutes.

In a bowl, beat egg and egg whites. Season with salt and pepper.

Heat the remaining ½ tablespoon oil in a skillet over medium-high heat. Add egg mixture, swirl to coat skillet, and cook for 1 to 2 minutes.

Add half of the filling, then fold omelet over filling. Spoon the last of the filling over the omelet and top with goat cheese.

Nutrition: 205 calories per serving, 13.5 grams protein, 7.3 grams carbohydrate, and 13.6 grams fat.

FAST-FUEL LUNCHES

Grilled Chicken and Vegetable Sandwich

MAKES 1 SERVING

3 ounces skinless boneless chicken breast
Salt
Black pepper
1 small zucchini, thinly sliced lengthwise
½ portobello mushroom, sliced ¼ inch thick
3 slices eggplant, ¼ inch thick
½ cup sliced red bell pepper
2 ounces French baguette
¼ cup spinach leaves

Heat the grill to high.

Season chicken with salt and black pepper. Grill chicken 3 to 4 minutes each side, or until done all the way through.

Season vegetables with salt and black pepper. Grill for 3 to 4 minutes, until softened.

Cut baguette in half. Top the baguette with spinach leaves. Then add grilled chicken breast and vegetables.

Nutrition: 393 calories per serving, 30.3 grams protein, 59.3 grams carbohydrate, and 3.9 grams fat.

Breaded Chicken with Green Beans

MAKES 1 SERVING

4 ounces skinless boneless chicken breast
¼ teaspoon salt
¼ teaspoon black pepper
¼ teaspoon garlic powder
¼ cup bread crumbs
16 green beans, ends trimmed
½ tablespoon olive oil
2 cloves garlic, minced

Preheat the oven to 400 degrees.

Season chicken with salt, pepper, and garlic powder. Coat chicken with bread crumbs and press bread crumbs into meat.

Bake chicken until golden brown, 16 to 20 minutes.

Bring small pot of water to boil over high heat. Add beans and cook for 5 to 6 minutes. Drain well.

Heat oil in a skillet over medium heat. Add garlic and green beans. Cook for 2 to 3 minutes. Season with salt and pepper.

Nutrition: 357 calories per serving, 29 grams protein, 28 grams carbohydrate, and 9.6 grams fat.

Note: To increase calories, increase serving size to 1½ servings.

Deli Turkey Pita Sandwich

MAKES 1 SERVING

1 whole-wheat pita
4 ounces thinly sliced deli turkey
1 small tomato, sliced
6 slices cucumber

½ avocado, sliced
2 lettuce leaves

Cut the pita bread in half. Fill it with turkey and vegetables.

Nutrition: 241 calories per serving, 22 grams protein, 51 grams carbohydrate, and 5 grams fat.

Salmon Barley Salad

MAKES 1 SERVING

3 ounces salmon
½ red bell pepper, seeded
6 asparagus spears
1 small zucchini, cut into round slices
1 tablespoon chopped flat-leaf parsley
½ teaspoon salt
¼ teaspoon black pepper
2 teaspoons lemon juice
½ teaspoon Dijon mustard
1 cup cooked barley
Lettuce leaves

Heat the grill to high. Grill salmon for 5 to 6 minutes. Cut salmon into 1-inch chunks.

Grill bell pepper, asparagus, and zucchini for 4 minutes, until vegetables are soft. Cut vegetables into 1-inch strips.

Place salmon and grilled vegetables in a bowl and toss with parsley, salt, black pepper, lemon juice, and mustard. Place cooked barley on lettuce leaves and top with the salmon and vegetables.

Nutrition: 418 calories per serving, 31.5 grams protein, 58 grams carbohydrate, and 6.7 grams fat.

Sautéed Shrimp and Citrus Salad

MAKES 1 SERVING

2 teaspoons olive oil
4 ounces peeled shrimp
Salt
Black pepper
1 orange, peeled and cut into sections
½ grapefruit, peeled and cut into sections
½ cup cherry tomatoes, cut in half
¼ cup sliced red onion
½ Gala apple, sliced
½ cup sliced cucumber
1 tablespoon chopped fresh mint

Heat 1 teaspoon oil in a skillet over medium-high heat. Season shrimp with salt and pepper. Sauté shrimp for 3 to 4 minutes.

In a large bowl, combine orange and grapefruit sections, tomatoes, onion, apple, cucumber, mint, and the remaining 1 teaspoon oil. Season with salt and pepper and toss.

Place fruit mixture on a plate and top with shrimp.

Nutrition: 393 calories per serving, 28 grams protein, 41 grams carbohydrate, and 13 grams fat.

Note: To increase calories, increase serving size to 1½ servings.

Tofu Singapore Noodles

MAKES 1 SERVING

¼ cup (2 ounces) rice vermicelli
1 teaspoon olive oil
¼ cup sliced onion
1 clove garlic, minced
¼ cup sliced red bell pepper
¼ cup sliced green bell pepper
4 ounces tofu
¼ cup bean sprouts
2 ounces seitan
3 tablespoon soy sauce
½ teaspoon black pepper
¼ teaspoon curry powder
1 green onion, chopped

Soak vermicelli in water for 20 minutes, then drain. Heat additional water in a pot over high heat and bring to a boil. Place vermicelli into boiling water and cook for 2 to 3 minutes. Drain.

Heat oil in a pan over medium-high heat. Add onion and garlic and cook for 1 to 2 minutes.

Add bell peppers, tofu, bean sprouts, and seitan. Cook for 3 to 4 minutes.

Add cooked vermicelli, soy sauce, black pepper, and curry powder. Cook for 2 to 3 minutes more.

Place in a bowl and sprinkle with chopped green onion.

Nutrition: 411 calories per serving, 33 grams protein, 36 grams carbohydrate, and 15 grams fat.

Note: To increase calories, increase serving size to 1½ servings.

Club Salad

MAKES 1 SERVING

¼ teaspoon salt
4 ounces skinless boneless chicken breast
2 cups chopped romaine lettuce
3 slices bacon, cooked
¼ avocado, chopped
¼ cup cherry tomatoes, cut in half
1 tablespoon balsamic vinegar
¼ teaspoon black pepper
⅛ teaspoon mustard
¼ teaspoon minced garlic
½ tablespoon olive oil

Fill a small pot halfway with water and bring to a simmer. Add salt and chicken; cook for 12 to 15 minutes, or until the internal temperature of the chicken reaches 160 degrees. Remove chicken to a plate, let cool, then cut into large cubes.

Mix chicken with remaining ingredients in a large bowl. Stir well to coat evenly.

Nutrition: 317 calories per serving, 29 grams protein, 21.3 grams carbohydrate, and 16.5 grams fat.

Grilled Chicken and Spinach

MAKES 1 SERVING

3 ounces skinless boneless chicken breast
1 tablespoon olive oil
¾ teaspoon salt
½ teaspoon black pepper
1 clove garlic, minced
1 zucchini, sliced
1 cup sliced mushrooms
1 cup spinach
1 tomato, peeled, seeded, and chopped

Preheat the grill. Rub chicken with ½ tablespoon oil, ½ teaspoon salt, and ¼ teaspoon pepper. Grill chicken for 7 to 8 minutes on each side, until cooked through.

Heat the remaining ½ tablespoon oil in a skillet over medium-high heat. Add garlic and sauté for 30 seconds. Add zucchini and mushrooms and sauté for 2 to 3 minutes. Add spinach, tomato, remaining ¼ teaspoon salt, and remaining ¼ teaspoon pepper. Cook for an additional 1 to 2 minutes and adjust seasonings. Serve vegetables with the chicken.

Nutrition: 258 calories per serving, 27 grams protein, 6 grams carbohydrate, and 14 grams fat.

Chicken Vegetable Soup

MAKES 1 SERVING

4 ounces skinless boneless chicken breast
½ tablespoon olive oil
1 clove garlic, minced
2 tablespoons chopped onion
½ teaspoon salt
½ teaspoon black pepper
½ cup chopped carrot
½ cup chopped tomato
½ cup green beans, cut into ½-inch pieces
½ cup chopped zucchini
16 ounces canned chicken broth
2 teaspoons poultry seasoning
Pinch chopped flat-leaf parsley

Sauté chicken in a small nonstick skillet over medium-high heat for 10 to 12 minutes, until cooked through. Remove from heat and cut into small cubes.

Heat oil in a small skillet over medium heat. Add garlic and onion. Sauté for 1 minute. Add chicken, salt, and pepper. Add carrot, tomato, green beans, zucchini, chicken broth, and poultry seasoning. Simmer for 20 minutes. Top with parsley before serving.

Nutrition: 310 calories per serving, 31 grams protein, 24 grams carbohydrate, and 10 grams fat.

Ahi Tuna Salad

MAKES 1 SERVING

4 ounces ahi tuna steak
Salt

Black pepper
1½ tablespoons olive oil
1 tablespoon lemon juice
¼ cup sliced radishes
½ cup sliced cucumber
1 cup mixed salad greens
¼ cup thinly sliced carrots

Season tuna with salt and pepper.

Heat ½ tablespoon oil in skillet over high heat. Cook tuna for 7 to 10 minutes, turning once. Do not overcook tuna; it should be pink in the center. Remove tuna from skillet and cut into thin slices.

In a large bowl, combine lemon juice, ¼ teaspoon salt, ¼ teaspoon pepper, and remaining 1 tablespoon oil. Mix well. Add radishes, cucumber, greens, and carrot; toss to coat.

Place the salad on the plate and arrange tuna slices on top.

Nutrition: 422 calories per serving, 28 grams protein, 30.5 grams carbohydrate, and 20 grams fat.

Broccoli Salad

MAKES 1 SERVING

2 cups broccoli florets
¼ teaspoon salt
¼ cup cherry tomatoes, cut in half
½ cup diced ham
¼ cup sliced red bell pepper
1 tablespoon red wine vinegar
½ tablespoon olive oil
¼ teaspoon black pepper
¼ teaspoon Dijon mustard

Fill a pot halfway with water and bring to a boil. Add broccoli and salt. Cook for 3 to 4 minutes. Drain broccoli and rinse with cold water.

Place broccoli in a large bowl, add all other ingredients, and mix well. Season with additional salt if needed.

Nutrition: 305 calories per serving, 15 grams protein, 18.5 grams carbohydrate, and 19 grams fat.

Note: To increase calories, increase the serving size to 1½ servings.

FAST-FUEL DINNERS

Chicken Fajitas

MAKES 1 SERVING

Salsa

1 small tomato, diced
½ jalapeño, diced
1 tablespoon chopped cilantro
1 tablespoon diced onion
1 teaspoon lime juice
½ teaspoon salt

Chicken Fajitas

4 ounces skinless boneless chicken breast, cut into ½-inch-thick strips
½ teaspoon lime juice
1 tablespoon plus ½ teaspoon olive oil
½ teaspoon salt
¼ teaspoon black pepper
¼ teaspoon chili powder
Pinch ground cumin

¼ teaspoon paprika
¼ teaspoon garlic powder
¼ teaspoon onion powder
½ red bell pepper, cut into thin strips
½ green bell pepper, cut into thin strips
½ yellow bell pepper, cut into thin strips
¼ onion, sliced
2 small flour tortillas
2 lime wedges

Combine salsa ingredients in a bowl and set aside.

Place chicken, lime juice, ½ teaspoon oil, salt, black pepper, chili powder, cumin, paprika, garlic powder, and onion powder in a separate bowl. Mix to coat well. Refrigerate for at least 20 minutes or up to 24 hours.

Heat ½ tablespoon oil in a skillet over medium-high heat. Add chicken strips and sauté for 5 to 6 minutes, until cooked through. Remove chicken from skillet and place on a plate.

In the same pan, heat the remaining ½ tablespoon oil. Add bell peppers and onion and sauté until tender. Remove mixture from pan.

Heat tortillas in the same pan until warm. Divide chicken and vegetable mixture between the tortillas and top with salsa.

Nutrition: 478 calories per serving, 32 grams protein, 47 grams carbohydrate, and 18 grams fat.

Note: To increase calories, increase serving size to 1½ servings.

Grilled Catfish with Coleslaw and Rice

MAKES 1 SERVING

Fish

3½ ounces catfish fillet
1 teaspoon olive oil
¼ teaspoon salt
¼ teaspoon black pepper
¼ teaspoon garlic powder
¼ teaspoon onion powder
¼ teaspoon paprika
¼ teaspoon chili powder
¼ teaspoon cayenne

Coleslaw

2 teaspoons rice vinegar
1 teaspoon sugar
¼ teaspoon salt
¼ teaspoon black pepper
1 cup finely shredded cabbage
¼ cup julienned carrots

Rice

¼ cup cooked rice
1 teaspoon chopped cilantro
Lemon wedges

To prepare the fish: Preheat the grill. Rub fish with oil and seasonings. Grill for 4 to 5 minutes on each side. The fish is done when it flakes with a fork.

To prepare the coleslaw: Combine rice vinegar, sugar, salt, and pepper in a bowl. Add the cabbage and carrot. Toss until well combined.

To prepare the rice: Mix rice with cilantro.

Serve grilled fish with coleslaw, rice, and lemon wedges.

Nutrition: 296 calories per serving, 25 grams protein, 23 grams carbohydrate, and 7 grams fat.

Seafood Mango Salad

MAKES 1 SERVING

4 ounces shrimp, peeled
2 ounces squid, bodies cut into ⅓-inch rings
½ cup sliced cucumber
½ cup sliced jicama
½ cup sliced mango
2 radishes, sliced
1 tablespoon lime juice
½ serrano chile, thinly sliced
1 tablespoon chopped cilantro

Bring a medium-sized pot of water to a boil over high heat. Boil shrimp and squid for 3 to 4 minutes, until cooked. Drain seafood.

Toss the other ingredients in a bowl. Add the seafood and serve.

Nutrition: 257 calories per serving, 36 grams protein, 26 grams carbohydrate, and 3 grams fat.

Note: To increase calories, increase the serving size to 1½ servings.

Hearty Steak and Potatoes

MAKES 1 SERVING

1 potato, peeled and cut into wedges
Salt
Black pepper
10 asparagus spears
4 ounces sirloin steak
½ tablespoon olive oil

Preheat the oven to 400 degrees. Line a baking sheet with parchment paper. Season the potato wedges with salt and pepper. Bake for 15 minutes. Place asparagus next to potato wedges and bake an additional 7 to 10 minutes, until vegetables are tender.

Rub steak with ¼ teaspoon salt and ¼ teaspoon pepper.

Heat oil in a skillet over high heat. Cook steak for 5 to 6 minutes on each side. Remove the steak to a plate and let sit for 5 minutes.

Serve steak with potato wedges and asparagus.

Nutrition: 435 calories per serving, 30 grams protein, 36 grams carbohydrate, and 19 grams fat.

Note: To increase calories, increase serving size to 1½ servings.

Sausage-Stuffed Zucchini with Orzo

MAKES 1 SERVING

½ Italian sausage link, casing removed
1 zucchini, halved lengthwise
1 Roma tomato, cut into 6 slices
Salt
Black pepper

2 tablespoons grated Parmesan cheese
2 ounces orzo

Heat a small pan over medium-high heat. Add the sausage and break it up with a spoon. Cook for 3 to 4 minutes, until no longer pink.

Preheat the oven to 350 degrees. Place zucchini on the baking sheet. Top zucchini with a layer of tomato slices and sausage, season with salt and pepper, and top with Parmesan. Bake for 20 minutes or until zucchini is tender.

Bring 2 quarts of salted water to a boil. Add orzo and boil for 9 minutes, until tender. Drain well.

Serve orzo with stuffed zucchini. Garnish with parsley.

Nutrition: 377 calories per serving, 17 grams protein, 48 grams carbohydrate, and 13 grams fat.
Note: To increase calories, increase the serving size to 1½ servings.

SLOW-FUEL DINNERS

Grilled Herb Chicken with Brussels Sprouts

MAKES 1 SERVING

4 ounces skinless boneless chicken breast
½ tablespoon olive oil
1 tablespoon chopped fresh rosemary
1 teaspoon chopped fresh thyme
Salt
Black pepper
1 cup Brussels sprouts, trimmed and cut in half lengthwise
½ cup cauliflower florets
1 tablespoon chopped flat-leaf parsley

Preheat the oven to 425 degrees.

Rub chicken with oil, rosemary, thyme, salt, and pepper. Set aside.

Season Brussels sprouts and cauliflower with salt and pepper. Place on a baking sheet and bake for 25 to 30 minutes.

Heat the grill. Oil the grill grate with paper towels. Using tongs, place chicken on the grill. Grill for 5 to 6 minutes on each side, until cooked through.

Serve grilled chicken with baked Brussels sprouts and cauliflower. Garnish with parsley.

Nutrition: 239 calories per serving, 13 grams fat, 24.8 grams carbohydrate, and 9.8 grams fat.

Note: To increase calories, increase serving size to 1½ servings.

Chicken and Vegetable Skewers

MAKES 1 SERVING

Sauce

1 teaspoon salt
½ teaspoon black pepper
1 clove garlic, minced
1 tablespoon olive oil
3 tablespoon chopped cilantro
1 teaspoon lime juice
½ teaspoon crushed red pepper

Chicken and Vegetables

3 ounces skinless boneless chicken breast, cut into 4 strips
½ red bell pepper, cut into 1½-inch pieces
½ green bell pepper, cut into 1½-inch pieces
4 mushrooms

½ red onion, cut into 4 wedges
½ zucchini, cut into ½-inch pieces

Prepare sauce: Combine all the sauce ingredients. Divide sauce between two bowls.

Prepare chicken and vegetables: Place the chicken strips in one of the bowls and coat with the sauce. Let sit for 10 minutes. Place vegetables in the other bowl and coat with sauce. Let sit for 10 minutes.

Soak 4 bamboo skewers in water for 10 minutes. Thread chicken strips on 2 skewers. Thread vegetables on 2 skewers. Discard remaining sauce. Grill chicken skewers and vegetable skewers for 6 to 8 minutes, until chicken is cooked through and vegetables are tender. Remove chicken and vegetables from skewers.

Nutrition: 263 calories per serving, 22 grams protein, 19 grams carbohydrate, and 11 grams fat.
Note: To increase calories, increase serving size to 1½ servings.

Naked Chicken Burrito

MAKES 1 SERVING

3 ounces grilled skinless boneless chicken breast
1 tablespoon olive oil
¾ teaspoon salt
¼ teaspoon black pepper
¼ teaspoon paprika
¼ teaspoon chili powder
¼ teaspoon onion powder
¼ teaspoon garlic powder
¼ can black beans
1 tomato, chopped

½ jalapeño, chopped
1 tablespoon chopped cilantro
1 tablespoon chopped onion
1 teaspoon lime juice
2 cups chopped romaine lettuce
3 slices avocado, chopped

Rub chicken with oil, ¼ teaspoon salt, pepper, paprika, chili powder, onion powder, and garlic powder.

Heat a griddle or skillet over medium-high heat and grill or sauté chicken breast for 8 to 9 minutes on each side, until done. Remove chicken from heat, let cool slightly, and chop.

Add black beans to a pot with a small amount of water. Simmer for 10 minutes and drain.

In a bowl combine tomato, jalapeño, cilantro, onion, lime juice, and the remaining ½ teaspoon salt. Set aside.

Place lettuce in a serving bowl. Add chicken, black beans, and avocado. Top with tomato mixture.

Nutrition: 405 calories per serving, 33 grams protein, 30 grams carbohydrate, and 17 grams fat.
Note: To increase calories, increase serving size to 1½ servings.

Grilled Flank Steak with Grilled Vegetable Salad

MAKES 1 SERVING

3 ounces flank steak
1¼ teaspoons salt
1¼ teaspoons black pepper
½ portobello mushroom
½ zucchini, sliced into ½-inch-thick rounds

½ green bell pepper, seeds removed
½ red bell pepper, seeds removed
3 slices eggplant, cut into ½-inch-thick strips
¼ red onion, thickly sliced
2 teaspoons olive oil
¼ teaspoon minced fresh rosemary
½ clove garlic, minced
1 teaspoon Dijon mustard
1 teaspoon balsamic vinegar

Season steak with ¼ teaspoon salt and ¼ teaspoon black pepper. Grill steak until desired doneness, 7 to 8 minutes for medium. Remove the steak to a plate and let rest for 5 minutes.

Grill mushroom, zucchini, bell peppers, eggplant, and onion until tender. Chop the vegetables.

In a large bowl whisk together 1 tablespoon water, oil, remaining 1 teaspoon salt, remaining 1 teaspoon black pepper, rosemary, garlic, mustard, and balsamic vinegar. Add vegetables and toss well.

Cut steak in strips and serve with vegetables.

Nutrition: 343 calories per serving, 23 grams protein, 20 grams carbohydrate, and 19 grams fat.

Pork Chop with Baby Broccoli

MAKES 1 SERVING

One 4-ounce pork chop
Salt
½ teaspoon black pepper
½ tablespoon olive oil
½ pound baby broccoli

Season pork chop with salt and pepper.

Heat oil in a skillet over medium heat. Cook pork chop for 6 to 7 minutes on each side, until cooked through.

Meanwhile, bring a pot of salted water to a boil. Add broccoli and cook for 3 to 4 minutes, until tender. Drain well and serve with pork chop.

Nutrition: 281 calories per serving, 27 grams protein, 14 grams carbohydrate, and 13 grams fat.
Note: To increase calories, increase serving size to 1½ servings.

Tri-Tip Sirloin Steak

MAKES 1 SERVING

Mashed Cauliflower

1 cup cauliflower
½ carrot, sliced
1 tablespoon milk
½ tablespoon butter
⅛ teaspoon salt
⅛ teaspoon black pepper

Mushroom Sauce

½ tablespoon butter
¼ teaspoon chopped garlic
1 teaspoon chopped onion
¼ cup sliced mushrooms
½ teaspoon cornstarch
¼ cup canned beef broth
½ teaspoon chopped flat-leaf parsley
⅛ teaspoon salt
¼ teaspoon black pepper

Steak

4 ounces tri-tip sirloin steak
¼ teaspoon salt
¼ teaspoon black pepper
½ tablespoon olive oil

Make mashed cauliflower: Fill a pot with 1½ cups water. Add cauliflower and carrot to the pot and cook over medium-high heat for 8 to 10 minutes. Drain and place cauliflower and carrot in a food processor. Add milk, butter, salt, and pepper. Process until smooth.

Make sauce: Melt butter in a small saucepan over medium-high heat. Add garlic, onion, and mushrooms. Sauté for 1 minute. Dissolve cornstarch in beef broth. Add broth to the saucepan and simmer for 3 to 4 minutes, until thick. Add parsley, salt, and pepper and stir well.

Make steak: Rub steak with salt and pepper. Heat pan over medium-high heat and add oil. Cook steak for 4 to 5 minutes on each side, until desired doneness.

Place steak on a plate and spoon sauce over it. Serve with mashed cauliflower.

Nutrition: 531 calories per serving, 26 grams protein, 16 grams carbohydrate, and 44 grams fat.

Egg Salad on Toast

MAKES 1 SERVING

2 eggs, boiled, peeled, and chopped
1 tablespoon mayonnaise
Black pepper
1 tablespoon finely chopped celery
¼ teaspoon Dijon mustard
1 piece of toast

Place eggs in a bowl. Add mayonnaise, dash of pepper, celery, and mustard and mix well.

Cut toast into two pieces. Scoop egg salad on each piece of toast.

Nutrition: 322 calories per serving, 16 grams protein, 16 grams carbohydrate, and 21.5 grams fat.
Note: To increase calories, increase serving size to 1½ servings.

Carrot Cake Protein Bites

MAKES 12 BITES

¾ cup unsweetened shredded coconut
6 Medjool dates, pitted
¾ cup walnuts or any kind of nuts
½ cup grated carrots
¼ cup protein powder

* All the smoothies count as fast-fuel snacks as well.

¼ cup unsweetened applesauce
1 teaspoon vanilla extract
1 teaspoon ground cinnamon
1 teaspoon ground nutmeg
¼ teaspoon ground cloves

Reserve ¼ cup of shredded coconut in a shallow dish for rolling. Place remaining ingredients in a food processor; process until fully combined. Form mixture into 1-inch balls and roll in reserved shredded coconut to coat completely. Refrigerate for a few hours or overnight, then serve. Keep chilled, or freeze in an airtight container. Will last for a few months.

Nutrition: 88 calories per bite, 3.5 grams protein, 12 grams carbohydrate, and 3 grams fat.

SLOW-FUEL SNACKS

Zucchini Pancakes with Smoked Salmon

MAKES 1 SERVING

1 zucchini, grated
1 egg
¼ teaspoon salt
¼ teaspoon black pepper
1 tablespoon flour
¼ tablespoon olive oil
2 ounces smoked salmon

In a bowl, combine grated zucchini, egg, salt, pepper, and flour.

Heat oil in a large skillet over medium heat. Spoon 3 tablespoons zucchini mixture onto skillet to make 1 pancake. Repeat with the remaining batter. Cook each pancake for 2 to 3 minutes on each side, until browned. Serve with smoked salmon.

Nutrition: 262 calories per serving, 20.5 grams protein, 13.5 grams carbohydrate, and 14 grams fat.
Note: To increase calories, increase serving size to 1½ servings.

Crab Salad on Avocado

MAKES 1 SERVING

½ cup crabmeat
1 tablespoon low-fat mayonnaise
Black pepper
Salt
½ avocado, pit removed
1 teaspoon sesame seeds, toasted

In a bowl, combine crabmeat and mayonnaise. Season with pepper and salt. Scoop crab salad on top of avocado. Sprinkle with sesame seeds.

Nutrition: 264 calories per serving, 8 grams protein, 8.5 grams carbohydrate, and 22 grams fat.
Note: To increase calories, increase serving size to 1½ servings.

Asparagus Wrapped with Deli Turkey

MAKES 1 SERVING

18 asparagus spears
6 slices deli turkey
Salt

Cut woody bottom off asparagus spears.

Fill a skillet with salted water and bring to a boil. Add asparagus and cook for 5 to 6 minutes; drain. Wrap a piece of turkey meat around 3 asparagus spears. Repeat with remainder of turkey and asparagus.

Nutrition: 212 calories per serving, 32 grams protein, 14 grams carbohydrate, and 3.1 grams fat.
Note: To increase calories, increase the recipe to 1½ servings.

Cucumber Cups

MAKES 1 SERVING

½ cucumber, cut in half lengthwise
2–3 ounces tuna, salmon, or hummus

With a spoon, scrape seeds out of cucumber halves. Stuff with tuna, salmon, or hummus.

Nutrition: With tuna: 89 calories per serving, 16 grams protein, 5.5 grams carbohydrate, and 1 gram fat. With hummus or salmon: 113 calories per serving, 5.5 grams protein, 14 grams carbohydrate, and 5 grams fat.
Note: If you stuff the cucumber with hummus, this recipe becomes a fast-fuel snack.

Fuelin' Veggie Juice

MAKES TWO 8-OUNCE SERVINGS

1 cup tightly packed kale or spinach
2 large tomatoes, cut into wedges
½ cucumber, sliced
1 large red bell pepper, seeded and cut into fourths
2 large stalks celery
1 large carrot

Working in the following order, process kale or spinach, tomatoes, cucumber, bell pepper, celery, and carrot through your juicer according to the manufacturer's directions.

Hoo-ya!

Preparing Quick, Delicious Food

I'm frequently time-crunched when it comes to food preparation. But I've learned some great shortcuts that not only shave time but boost flavor. Here's a rundown.

Vegetables

- Sprinkle fresh herbs over vegetables before you roast, stir-fry, or steam them.
- Broil sliced veggies like zucchini, bell peppers, eggplant, and tomatoes until they turn slightly brown around the edges. Serve warm topped with no-sugar-added marinara sauce.
- Sauté zucchini, eggplant, onions, mushrooms, and so forth in a couple of tablespoons of olive oil until tender. Serve over whole-wheat pasta for a quick pasta primavera.
- Microwave fresh or frozen vegetables and sprinkle them with a little garlic, onion, or herbs such as rosemary or thyme for a burst of flavor.

- Stir chopped fresh spinach or kale and crushed walnuts into steamed brown rice.
- Chop up veggies on the weekend and store them in the fridge. Cut up a batch of bell peppers, carrots, or broccoli. You can enjoy them on a salad or as a quick snack.
- Toss steamed broccoli florets and tomatoes with whole-grain pasta, minced garlic, and a little olive oil.
- Combine cooked couscous with chopped mint, scallions, and olive oil.

Fruits

- Add sliced grapes, chopped apples, or chopped pears to a chicken salad made with low-fat or fat-free mayonnaise.
- Toss some whole blueberries into a salad, or sweeten up sliced strawberries with a little honey.
- Snack on frozen red grapes for a sweet treat.
- Keep a supply of frozen berries on hand to toss into smoothies or on cereal.

Meats and Fish

- Top broiled lean meat, chicken, or fish with salsa.
- Poach salmon in an infusion of green tea and ginger.
- Spray meat, poultry, or fish with a little olive oil cooking spray prior to baking, broiling, or grilling to bring out the flavors.
- Marinate meat, poultry, or fish in low-fat Italian salad dressing prior to cooking to enhance tenderness.

CHAPTER 9

MEATLESS FUELING

I frequently hear from vegans and vegetarians wanting to know whether they can follow the Body Fuel plan while at the same time not eating animal proteins. My answer: you bet, and I'll show you how here. Personally, I'm a meat eater and always have been, but I try to eat as many plant foods as I possibly can because of their tremendous nutritional worth. Vegetarians and vegans know this, and they're usually super-healthy as a result. A plant-based diet is an excellent way to eat. Plus, as long as the world is populated with vegans and vegetarians, well, that's more rib-eyes for me.

There are various types of "plant eaters," from vegans who eat no animal products whatsoever to folks who don't eat chicken or beef but might enjoy some fish now and then (sometimes called pescetarians). If you're in the vegan crowd, your diet consists of soy foods, beans and legumes, grains, fruits, vegetables, nuts, and seeds. You get your protein from soy, beans, legumes, nuts, and seeds. It's best for you to focus on beans and legumes as your chief sources of protein, since nuts are high in calories for such little packages. You'd probably pack on pounds if you ate too many nuts.

There are really different types of vegetarians:

Semi-vegetarian. You eat dairy, egg products, poultry, and fish but avoid red meat. If you're in this category, the regular Body Fuel plan will work for you easily. You'll want to try to eat more poultry and fish, and because you have no problem with eggs, eat more of those, too. So where I call for red meat, pork, veal, or lamb, simply substitute any of the other proteins, such as poultry or fish.

Lacto-ovo. You eat eggs and dairy products but avoid poultry, fish, and red meat. While following the Body Fuel plan, you can include eggs as a protein source, but you'll get most of your other protein from beans, legumes, nuts, and seeds. My plan contains small amounts of dairy that can be cut out by substituting with nondairy milks.

Lacto. You eat dairy but avoid all other animal products and eggs. To follow the Body Fuel plan, I suggest that you substitute nondairy products for the dairy you usually include. You'll get better results that way.

Beyond these definitions, if you want to improve your vegan or vegetarian diet and adapt it to the Body Fuel plan, do the following:

Focus on the plant proteins you can eat. As I've mentioned previously, protein is the key element for muscle growth, recovery, fat burning, and appetite control. Vegans and vegetarians who work out and want to lose weight should include plants that offer quality proteins, which I've listed in the "Hoo-ya" on page 162. My smoothies are made with plant-based protein powder, so these are perfect for a meatless diet.

Also, tofu is a terrific choice for a vegan diet. There are different types and brands of tofu on the market. You have to sample different types to find out which ones you prefer. Tofu is unique in that it picks up the flavor of whatever it's cooked with. It tastes really great when substituted for animal proteins in Italian and Asian dishes.

Hoo-ya!

Quality Plant-Based Proteins

Almonds
Almond butter
Black beans, cooked
Black-eyed peas, cooked
Cashews
Chickpeas, cooked
Edamame
Hemp seeds
Hummus
Kidney beans, cooked
Lentils, cooked
Lima beans, cooked
Nondairy cheeses
Nondairy yogurt, plain
Peanut butter
Peas, cooked
Pinto beans, cooked
Plant-based protein powders
Portobello mushrooms
Pumpkin seeds
Quinoa, cooked
Seitan
Sunflower seeds
Tempeh
Textured vegetable protein (TVP), cooked
Tofu
Veggie baked beans
Veggie burger
Veggie dog

Balance your slow fuels and fast fuels, according to the blocks. You can eat slow fuels liberally because they include all low-calorie, high-fiber vegetables. Refer to page 33 for a complete list. As for fast fuels, these include fruits and higher-starch vegetables—perfect for a plant-based, meatless diet. Eat the proper number of fast fuels for the corresponding block you're on: four daily fast fuels on Block 3, two daily fast fuels on Block 2, and one daily fast fuel on Block 1. All of these fuels are crucial for the growth and development of muscles.

Take in fat naturally. You'll get good fats automatically by eating nuts and seeds. As with the regular Body Fuel plan, include a tablespoon a day of olive oil, coconut oil, or flaxseed oil, if desired.

Watch your liquids and refined foods. Don't drink your calories in the form of sugary drinks or commercial juice. Stick to water, and drink plenty of it. Avoid refined sugar, including high-fructose corn syrup, cane sugar, and so many others. Don't ingest obviously fake foods like aspartame, other fake sugars, food colorings, or other ingredients you aren't familiar with.

Go organic. Organic foods have more nutrients and fewer toxins in them. Eat whole, unadulterated foods in general—not processed foods from a box or can with a zillion ingredients in them.

If you do all of these things—heck, if everyone did all of these things—we would all be much fitter and healthier.

In the section below, I'm giving you sample menus for meatless Body Fuel meals. You'll find a one-week sample for Block 3, a one-week sample for Block 2, and a one-week sample for Block 1.

SAMPLE MEATLESS BODY FUEL PLANS

BLOCK 3

BLOCK 3 • DAY 1

Breakfast (Fast Fuel)

1¼ cups packaged cereal such as Special K or a high-fiber cereal like raisin bran or Fiber One

1 tablespoon hemp seeds (protein) to sprinkle over your cereal

1 cup almond milk for the cereal

Lunch (Fast Fuel)

Chicken Vegetable Soup (replace the chicken in the recipe on page 140 with ½ to 1 cup canned kidney beans for a delicious meatless soup)

1 medium apple

Dinner (Fast Fuel)

1 or 2 portobello mushrooms, sautéed in 1 tablespoon olive oil

Steamed asparagus

1 baked potato, topped with 1–2 tablespoons dairy-free sour cream, if desired

Snack 1 (Fast Fuel)

Island Breeze Smoothie

Snack 2

½ cup hummus

Baby carrots for dipping

BLOCK 3 • DAY 2

Breakfast (Fast Fuel)

Oatmeal with Berries

1 tablespoon hemp seeds to sprinkle over your oatmeal

Lunch (Fast Fuel)

Vegetable wraps: alfalfa sprouts, cucumber slices, tomato slices, and 2 slices avocado in a flour tortilla spread with 2–3 tablespoons hummus

Dinner (Fast Fuel)

Pinto beans (1 cup for men, ½ cup for women)

Kale sautéed in 1 tablespoon olive oil

Brown rice, cooked (1 cup for men, ½ cup for women)

Snack 1

Handful of almonds

8 ounces *Fuelin' Veggie Juice*

Snack 2 (Fast Fuel)

Bananafana Cocoa Smoothie

BLOCK 3 • DAY 3

Breakfast (Fast Fuel)

Scrambled Eggs with Tomatoes and Potatoes (if you don't eat eggs, replace the eggs in this recipe with tofu)

Lunch (Fast Fuel)

Chicken Vegetable Soup (replace the chicken in the recipe on page 140 with ½ to 1 cup canned kidney beans for a delicious meatless soup)

1 orange

Dinner (Fast Fuel)

Chickpeas (1 cup for men, ½ cup for women) on a bed of mixed salad greens, drizzled with low-fat salad dressing

Whole-grain or sprouted-grain bread (2 slices for men, 1 slice for women)

Snack 1

Handful of almonds

Raw cut-up slow-fuel veggies

Snack 2 (Fast Fuel)

Island Breeze Smoothie

BLOCK 3 • DAY 4

Breakfast (Fast Fuel)

Cooked quinoa (1 cup for men, ½ cup for women), sweetened with a little cinnamon and honey

½ grapefruit

Lunch (Fast Fuel)

Mixed greens and salad vegetables topped with cubed tofu (1 cup for men, ½ cup for women) and drizzled with 1 tablespoon olive oil and 1 tablespoon balsamic vinegar

1 apple

Dinner (Fast Fuel)

Veggie burger, pan-fried

1 cup stewed tomatoes

Brown rice, cooked (1 cup for men, ½ cup for women)

Snack 1

Handful of almonds

Assorted chopped raw vegetables

Snack 2 (Fast Fuel)

Egg Salad on Toast (if you don't eat eggs, replace the eggs in this recipe with tofu)

BLOCK 3 • DAY 5

Breakfast (Fast Fuel)

Mango Tango Smoothie

Lunch (Fast Fuel)

Caesar salad with 2 ounces shredded nondairy cheese, romaine lettuce, and green bell pepper strips with 1–2 tablespoons low-fat Caesar salad dressing

Whole-grain or sprouted-grain bread (2 slices for men, 1 slice for women)

Dinner (Fast Fuel)

Tofu Singapore Noodles

Snack 1 (Fast Fuel)

Handful of almonds

1 peach or other seasonal fruit

Snack 2

Cucumber Cups (stuffed with hummus)

BLOCK 3 • DAY 6

Breakfast (Fast Fuel)

1 cup nondairy yogurt

1 cup fresh berries

Lunch (Fast Fuel)

Leftover *Tofu Singapore Noodles*

Dinner (Fast Fuel)

1 cup chopped cooked portobello mushrooms, mixed with no-sugar-added marinara sauce and served over cooked whole-wheat pasta (1 cup for men, ½ cup for women)

Snack 1

Sliced cucumbers dipped in hummus (1 cup for men, ½ cup for women)

Snack 2 (Fast Fuel)

Bananafana Cocoa Smoothie

BLOCK 3 • DAY 7

Breakfast (Fast Fuel)

2 veggie sausage patties, pan-fried

1 Roma tomato, sliced

Grits, cooked (1 cup for men, ½ cup for women)

Lunch (Fast Fuel)

Organic lentil soup, canned (2 cups for men, 1 cup for women)

Whole-grain or sprouted-grain bread (2 slices for men, 1 slice for women)

Dinner (Fast Fuel)

Veggie burger, pan-fried

1 cup stewed tomatoes

1 baked potato, topped with 1–2 tablespoons dairy-free sour cream, if desired

Snack 1

2 ounces nondairy cheese

1 cup kale chips

Snack 2 (Fast Fuel)

Mango Tango Smoothie

SAMPLE SHOPPING LIST FOR BLOCK 3—MEATLESS

Vegetables

Potatoes

Kale

Asparagus

Baby carrots (for snacking)

Alfalfa sprouts

Bean sprouts

Cucumbers

Roma tomatoes

Tomatoes, such as beefsteak
Mixed salad greens
Romaine lettuce
Bell peppers: red and green
Spinach
Onions
Garlic
Green onions
Carrots
Green beans
Zucchini
Broccoli
Cauliflower
Flat-leaf parsley
Celery

Fruits

Apples
Berries
Avocados
Oranges
Grapefruit
Peaches
Bananas

Plant-Based Proteins

Portobello mushrooms
Hemp seeds
Hummus
Vanilla plant-based protein powder
Chocolate plant-based protein powder
Raw almonds
Tofu
Quinoa
Veggie burgers
Nondairy cheese
Nondairy yogurt
Veggie sausage patties
Seitan

Cereals, Grains, and Bread

Packaged cereal such as Special K or a high-fiber cereal like raisin bran or Fiber One
Oatmeal
Flour tortillas
Brown rice
Whole-grain or sprouted-grain bread
Whole-wheat pasta
Grits
Vermicelli

Frozen Foods

Frozen peaches
Frozen mango

Canned Goods

Kidney beans
Pinto beans
Stewed tomatoes
Chickpeas
Organic lentil soup
Unsweetened pineapple chunks (drain and freeze for smoothies)

Oils and Vinegar

Olive oil
Balsamic vinegar
Almond butter
Mayonnaise

Spices

Cinnamon
Curry powder

Condiments and Sweetening Agents

Low-fat salad dressing
Dairy-free sour cream
Soy sauce
Low-fat Caesar salad dressing
No-sugar-added marinara sauce
Vegetable broth (in a box)
Honey
Raw organic agave syrup

Beverages

Almond milk, unsweetened

Miscellaneous

Kale chips
Chia seeds
Flaxseeds

BLOCK 2

BLOCK 2 • DAY 1

Breakfast (Fast Fuel)

1¼ cups packaged cereal such as Special K or a high-fiber cereal like raisin bran or Fiber One

1 tablespoon hemp seeds to sprinkle over your cereal

1 cup almond milk for the cereal

Lunch (Fast Fuel)

2 tablespoons almond butter spread on 1 slice whole-grain bread

Organic vegetarian vegetable soup, canned (2 cups for men, 1 cup for women)

Dinner

1 or 2 portobello mushrooms, sautéed in 1 tablespoon olive oil

Steamed asparagus

Snack 1

Handful of almonds

Assorted raw slow-fuel vegetables

Snack 2

½ cup hummus

Baby carrots for dipping

BLOCK 2 • DAY 2

Breakfast (Fast Fuel)

Very Berry Smoothie

Lunch (Fast Fuel)

Vegetable wraps: alfalfa sprouts, cucumber slices, tomato slices, and 2 slices of avocado in a flour tortilla spread with 2–3 tablespoons hummus

Dinner

Faux chicken strips (1 cup for men, ½ cup for women) stir-fried with slow-fuel stir-fry vegetables, soy sauce, and 1–2 tablespoons olive oil

Snack 1

Handful of almonds

8 ounces *Fuelin' Veggie Juice*

Snack 2

Handful of pumpkin seeds

1 cup almond milk

BLOCK 2 • DAY 3

Breakfast (Fast Fuel)

Scrambled Eggs with Tomatoes and Potatoes (if you don't eat eggs, replace the eggs in this recipe with tofu)

Lunch

Organic vegan chili, canned (2 cups for men, 1 cup for women)

Dinner

Chickpeas (1 cup for men, ½ cup for women) on a bed of mixed salad greens, drizzled with low-fat salad dressing

Snack 1

Handful of almonds

Raw cut-up slow fuel veggies

Snack 2 (Fast Fuel)

Island Breeze Smoothie

BLOCK 2 • DAY 4

Breakfast (Fast Fuel)

Cooked quinoa (1 cup for men, ½ cup for women), sweetened with a little cinnamon and honey

½ grapefruit

Lunch (Fast Fuel)

Mixed greens and salad vegetables topped with cubed tofu (1 cup for men, ½ cup for women), drizzled with 1 tablespoon olive oil and 1 tablespoon balsamic vinegar.

1 apple

Dinner

Veggie burger, pan-fried

1 cup stewed tomatoes

Snack 1

Handful of almonds

Assorted chopped raw vegetables

Snack 2

Cucumber Cups (stuffed with hummus)

BLOCK 2 • DAY 5

Breakfast (Fast Fuel)

Mango Tango Smoothie

Lunch

Caesar salad with 2 ounces shredded nondairy cheese, romaine lettuce, and green bell pepper strips with 1–2 tablespoons low-fat Caesar salad dressing

Dinner (Fast Fuel)

Tofu Singapore Noodles

Snack 1

Handful of pumpkin seeds

1 cup almond milk

Snack 2

1 cup organic vegetarian vegetable soup, canned

BLOCK 2 • DAY 6

Breakfast (Fast Fuel)

1 cup nondairy yogurt

1 cup fresh berries

Lunch (Fast Fuel)

Leftover *Tofu Singapore Noodles*

Dinner

1 cup chopped cooked portobello mushrooms, mixed with no-sugar-added marinara sauce and served over strips of sautéed zucchini

Snack 1

Sliced cucumbers dipped in hummus (1 cup for men, ½ cup for women)

Snack 2

Handful of almonds

Assorted raw cut-up slow-fuel vegetables

BLOCK 2 • DAY 7

Breakfast (Fast Fuel)

2 veggie sausage patties, pan-fried

1 Roma tomato, sliced

Grits, cooked (1 cup for men, ½ cup for women)

Lunch

Organic lentil soup, canned (2 cups for men, 1 cup for women)

Dinner

Veggie burger, pan-fried

1 cup stewed tomatoes

Snack 1

2 ounces nondairy cheese

1 cup kale chips

Snack 2 (Fast Fuel)

Bananafana Cocoa Smoothie

SAMPLE SHOPPING LIST FOR BLOCK 2—MEATLESS

Vegetables

Potatoes
Asparagus
Cucumbers
Roma tomatoes
Tomatoes, such as beefsteak
Broccoli
Cauliflower
Bell peppers: red and green
Spinach
Zucchini
Celery

Fruits

Berries
Bananas

Plant-Based Proteins

Hemp seeds
Almond butter
Portobello mushrooms
Pumpkin seeds
Hummus
Vanilla plant-based protein powder
Chocolate plant-based protein powder
Tofu
Nondairy cheese
Nondairy yogurt

Cereals, Grains, and Bread

Packaged cereal such as Special K or a high-fiber cereal like raisin bran or Fiber One

Canned Goods

Organic vegetarian vegetable soup
Organic vegan chili
Stewed tomatoes
Chickpeas
Organic lentil soup
Unsweetened pineapple chunks (drain and freeze for smoothies)

Beverages

Almond milk, unsweetened

Miscellaneous

Kale chips

BLOCK 1

BLOCK 1 • DAY 1

Breakfast (Fast Fuel)

1¼ cups packaged cereal such as Special K or a high-fiber cereal like raisin bran or Fiber One

1 tablespoon hemp seeds to sprinkle over your cereal

1 cup almond milk for the cereal

Lunch

2 tablespoons almond butter spread on celery sticks

Organic vegetarian vegetable soup, canned (2 cups for men, 1 cup for women)

Dinner

1 or 2 portobello mushrooms, sautéed in 1 tablespoon olive oil

Steamed asparagus

Snack 1

Handful of almonds

Assorted raw slow-fuel vegetables

Snack 2

½ cup hummus

Baby carrots for dipping

BLOCK 1 • DAY 2

Breakfast (Fast Fuel)

Mango Tango Smoothie

Lunch

Vegetable wraps: alfalfa sprouts, cucumber slices, tomato slices, and 2 slices of avocado wrapped in lettuce leaves with 2–3 tablespoons hummus

Dinner

Faux chicken strips (1 cup for men, ½ cup for women) stir-fried with slow-fuel stir-fry vegetables, soy sauce, and 1–2 tablespoons olive oil

Snack 1

Handful of almonds

8 ounces *Fuelin' Veggie Juice*

Snack 2

Handful of pumpkin seeds

1 cup almond milk

BLOCK 1 • DAY 3

Breakfast (Fast Fuel)

Scrambled Eggs with Tomatoes and Potatoes (if you don't eat eggs, replace the eggs in this recipe with tofu)

Lunch

Organic vegan chili, canned (2 cups for men, 1 cup for women)

Dinner

Chickpeas (1 cup for men, ½ cup for women) on a bed of mixed salad greens, drizzled with low-fat salad dressing

Snack 1

Handful of almonds

Raw cut-up slow-fuel veggies

Snack 2

Cucumber Cups (stuffed with hummus)

BLOCK 1 • DAY 4

Breakfast (Fast Fuel)

Cooked quinoa (1 cup for men, ½ cup for women), sweetened with a little cinnamon and honey

½ grapefruit

Lunch

Mixed greens and salad vegetables topped with cubed tofu (1 cup for men, ½ cup for women), drizzled with 1 tablespoon olive oil and 1 tablespoon balsamic vinegar

Dinner

Veggie burger, pan-fried

1 cup stewed tomatoes

Snack 1

Handful of almonds

Assorted chopped raw vegetables

Snack 2

Cucumber Cups (stuffed with hummus)

BLOCK 1 • DAY 5

Breakfast

1 cup nondairy yogurt

Lunch

Caesar salad with 2 ounces shredded nondairy cheese, romaine lettuce, and green bell pepper strips with 1–2 tablespoons low-fat Caesar salad dressing

Dinner (Fast Fuel)

Tofu Singapore Noodles

Snack 1

Handful of pumpkin seeds

1 cup almond milk

Snack 2

1 cup organic vegetarian vegetable soup, canned

BLOCK 1 • DAY 6

Breakfast

Tofu scrambled with chopped tomatoes, onions, and green bell pepper slices in 1 tablespoon olive oil

Lunch (Fast Fuel)

Leftover *Tofu Singapore Noodles*

Dinner

1 cup chopped cooked portobello mushrooms, mixed with no-sugar-added marinara sauce and served over strips of sautéed zucchini

Snack 1

Sliced cucumbers dipped in hummus (1 cup for men, ½ cup for women)

Snack 2

Handful of almonds

Assorted raw cut-up slow-fuel vegetables

BLOCK 1 • DAY 7

Breakfast

2 veggie sausage patties, pan-fried

1 Roma tomato, sliced

Lunch

Organic lentil soup, canned (2 cups for men, 1 cup for women)

Dinner

Veggie burger, pan-fried

1 cup stewed tomatoes

Snack 1

2 ounces nondairy cheese

1 cup kale chips

Snack 2 (Fast Fuel)

Bananafana Cocoa Smoothie

SAMPLE SHOPPING LIST FOR BLOCK 1—MEATLESS

Vegetables

Asparagus

Baby carrots

Cucumbers

Roma tomato

Tomatoes, such as beefsteak

Broccoli
Cauliflower
Bell peppers: red and green
Romaine lettuce
Lettuce, such as iceberg or buttercrunch
Alfalfa sprouts
Spinach or kale
Mixed salad greens
Zucchini
Celery
Onions

Fruits

Bananas
Avocados
Grapefruit

Plant-Based Proteins

Portobello mushrooms
Faux chicken strips
Hummus
Tofu
Nondairy cheese
Nondairy yogurt

Frozen Foods

Frozen stir-fry vegetables

Canned Goods

Organic vegetarian vegetable soup
Stewed tomatoes
Chickpeas

There's no enigmatic alchemy underlying successful vegetarian and vegan menu planning and cooking. All you need is some nutritional know-how, a little spark of imagination, and a spirit of exploration to get started. And look to vegetarian and vegan cookbooks for inspiration. The ruling principles are simple enough to execute: serve a variety of foods, focus on vegetarian proteins, distinguish between slow- and fast-fuel carbs, and be sure the meal is filling. So pull up the meat anchor and open yourself up to a world of menu ideas.

Hoo-ya!

Creative Meatless Cooking

It's not that difficult to create fabulous—and healthful—meatless meals. Here are some ideas to help you.

Cook up meatless versions of your favorite meat-containing dishes. Substitute veggies such as cooked spinach, green peppers, zucchini, eggplant, and onions for the ground beef in your favorite lasagna and serve it up with a salad of mixed greens. Take out the beef in chili and replace it with black beans or kidney beans, or even textured vegetable protein. You'll never even taste the difference.

Enjoy ethnic cuisines. Did you know that most of the world eats a largely vegetarian diet? It's true. Think about it. Asian countries have transformed mixed vegetables into delicious stir-fries, mostly meatless. Do this yourself: toss in cubes of tofu, tempeh, or seitan in place of meat. Then serve your stir-fry over brown rice for a meal that's both delicious and filling.

A lot of Italian dishes can be transformed into vegetarian meals, too. Top spaghetti with tofu and marinara sauce. Use tofu as a substitute for ricotta cheese in lasagna or stuffed shells.

Look to Middle Eastern and Latin cuisines for delicious meatless meals. If you like Mexican food, you're in luck—a meatless Mexican meal can be put together easily from tortillas, beans (whole or mashed), avocado, and salsa.

Devour soups and salads. Neither really needs meat. A hearty soup made with beans or lentils can be a satisfying main dish. Few people can tell the difference between a meat-based chili and a vegetarian chili when it's spiced right. Serve the soup or chili with a salad to complete the meal.

CHAPTER 10

FUEL TOOLS: BODY FUEL SUPPLEMENTS

I'm frequently asked about nutritional supplements—what to take and, just as important, what not to take. After all, supplements are everywhere: health food stores, pharmacies, supermarkets, and the Internet. Many of these products claim to boost, cleanse, enhance, or otherwise benefit every body system you can imagine. Millions of Americans take them.

If you're among the supplemented masses, how do you know you're taking the right ones? Should you add in that super-duper fat-burning supplement you just read about on the Internet? What about that latest, greatest natural hormone booster everyone is blogging about?

I'll give you my take on supplements and how I personally approach the issue. Let's start with multivitamin/mineral supplements, otherwise known as the "multi," probably the most ubiquitous of the bunch.

MY ADVICE ON MULTIS

These supplements are touted as a way to help prevent chronic diseases. But honestly, no one really knows for sure if this far-reaching claim is true. The government even requires a disclaimer on all supplement labels, saying that the product in question "is not intended to treat, cure, or prevent any disease."

For multivitamin/mineral supplements, the United States Preventive Services Task Force, an independent panel that issues recommendations on preventive health care, stated that there's little proof that supplemental vitamins have any benefit for the prevention of two big killers, heart disease and cancer. Their conclusions were reported in the *Annals of Internal Medicine* in 2013.

The task force came down hard on vitamin E and beta-carotene, previously believed to help prevent cancer and heart disease. Research on these supplements has shown that neither works for prevention. Beta-carotene, in particular, was found to actually amplify the odds of lung cancer in at-risk populations (smokers, for example).

So, to take vitamin/mineral supplements or to not take them? This is a very confusing question, and the complete story isn't in yet. Personally, I don't even take a multi. Here's why: I eat a wide range of whole foods, including vegetables, some fruit, meat, chicken, fish, beans, grains, nuts, and seeds. Plus, I love to juice, which is like drinking a full glass of vitamins and minerals. So basically, I eat real foods that are endowed by nature with nutrients. I get all the vitamins and minerals I need directly from those foods.

I side with the health professionals who say that *most* dietary supplements are no substitute for a healthful lifestyle. A problem with taking multivitamins is that it may lead you to think you don't need to do the other lifestyle things that are important but may be hard, such as following a good diet, exercising, or quitting smoking. Unfortunately, people seem to want a magic pill or a quick fix. Dietary supplements are neither.

Selecting a variety of nutritious foods should provide the essential nutrients we need for good health. You'll obtain those nutrients from the Magnificent 7 on the Body Fuel plan. Take a look at the following box and you'll see the vitamins supplied by my plan.

Hoo-ya!

Vitamins and Minerals

Vitamins are directly involved in the metabolism of carbohydrates, proteins, and fats. You'll get the following vitamins on my plan:

Vitamin A: green leafy vegetables, carrots, fruits, eggs
B vitamins: protein foods, whole grains, legumes, fruits, vegetables
Vitamin C: fruits and vegetables
Vitamin D: fish
Vitamin E: whole grains, green leafy vegetables, nuts and seeds, eggs

Minerals also play a role in metabolism, and they are building blocks for bone, cartilage, and teeth. The Body Fuel plan provides the following minerals:

Iron: meats, poultry, eggs, nuts, green leafy vegetables, fruits
Calcium: salmon, green leafy vegetables, broccoli, calcium-fortified almond milk
Copper: meats, shellfish, nuts
Magnesium: meats, nuts
Phosphorus: meats, poultry, fish, nuts
Potassium: fruits, vegetables
Selenium: whole grains, fish, eggs
Zinc: shellfish, meats, whole grains, vegetables

I also agree with health experts that there are certain populations who may need vitamin and mineral supplements: pregnant women, the elderly, strict vegans, or people who might be chronically ill, for example. And certainly, many women suffer deficiencies in calcium and sometimes iron.

Also, some people who live in northern climates or who have very dark skin might need to take supplemental vitamin D_3. One of the chief sources of this vitamin is sunlight. When the sun's UVB rays hit your skin, a chemical reaction occurs, and your body begins converting a hormone in the skin into vitamin D. People who live in less sunny areas are thus often at risk of a vitamin D deficiency because of limited sun exposure. So are dark-skinned individuals, because their skin does not absorb UVB rays well.

If you fall into any of these at-risk groups, you may need to supplement. There's just no simple, one-size-fits-all approach. It depends on the individual and what a physician might recommend—so definitely check with your doctor.

THE HYPE ON FAT BURNERS AND MUSCLE BUILDERS

Here's an area where you need to be on your toes: supplements that claim to burn fat or build muscle. There's so much hype here that it defies rationality. A good place to start cutting through the crap is to consult the Food and Drug Administration's website, www.fda.gov, on which the FDA has exposed nearly three hundred fraudulent products—marketed mainly for weight loss and muscle building, as well as for sexual enhancement. These products have been found to contain prescription drug ingredients, synthetic steroids, or other hidden or deceptively labeled ingredients—many of which can be dangerous, especially when taken unknowingly. In fact, the FDA has reported incidents of serious and even life-threatening side effects associated with the use of these products, including heart and circulation problems, liver damage, kidney failure, and death.

So be a smart consumer and protect yourself. As advised by the FDA, beware of any dietary supplement that:

- Claims to be an "alternative to FDA-approved drugs" or that advertises benefits you might get from taking prescription drugs
- Purports to be a legal or natural alternative to anabolic steroids
- Contains a warning label that if you take the supplement, "you may test positive in drug tests"
- Promises extreme, exaggerated results like "quick and effective," "cure-all," "can treat or cure diseases," or "totally safe," or features

far-fetched "testimonials" about "amazing" results from taking the supplement in question
- Sounds too good to be true

Another source for tracking down the reliability of supplements is Consumer Lab.com, a supplement-testing company. Since 1999, this independent laboratory has been rigorously testing vitamins, minerals, herbal supplements, and other items and has uncovered much evidence that a lot of supplements don't always contain the ingredients and substances listed on their labels.

Ultimately, for us consumers it's caveat emptor—let the buyer beware—when it comes to dietary supplements.

SUPPLEMENTS WITH MERIT

That said, I am not against all supplements. There are a few that I do recommend. The reason is that they are more like actual food than processed pills, or they've been well validated by science for their nutritional necessity. The following supplements are strictly optional on Body Fuel, but I do feel they have merits. Here's a rundown.

Green Powders

Nearly every credible health expert or organization recommends that we eat at least five servings of produce each day to get the nutrients required for good health. But what if you're not a big vegetable eater? Supplement with green powders. These superfoods are green veggies in concentrated form and thus a great way to fill in the nutritional blanks. They're packed with all the vitamins and minerals you find in fruits and vegetables: beta-carotene, B vitamins, vitamin C, calcium, magnesium, selenium, and more.

Made from organic grasses, green powders have a sweet, slightly grassy, wheaty flavor. You stir or blend them into a liquid and drink it down. I add the powder to any homemade juice or smoothie. Besides the powdered form, this supplement comes in liquids, tablets, and capsules.

Each green powder has its own set of nutritional payoffs. Here's a quick look:

- *Spirulina.* This micro-algae is naturally high in vitamin A, amino acids, and disease-preventing antioxidants. Spirulina supplies gamma-linolenic acid (GLA), an omega-6 fat being studied for its cancer-fighting properties. If you're a vegan or a vegetarian, spirulina is a great source of vitamin B_{12}, normally found only in foods of animal origin.
- *Chlorella.* Here's another micro-algae that also contains vitamin A, vitamin B_{12}, and amino acids. It is particularly high in chlorophyll, considered a blood booster because its makeup is very similar to the oxygen-carrying hemoglobin found in red blood cells. Many health care practitioners believe that supplementing with chlorophyll is a good way to raise red cell blood count, increase circulation, strengthen immunity, and help improve digestion.
- *Alfalfa.* This plant is a legume that is packed with the minerals potassium and calcium, plus the B vitamin niacin, which is helpful in normalizing cholesterol and reducing artery-clogging plaque.
- *Wheatgrass and barley grass.* Wheatgrass is a nutritional powerhouse of twenty-two different vitamins. If you have a wheat allergy, you can consume wheatgrass safely, since it doesn't contain any of the gluten found in wheat and its relatives. Barley grass is rich is protein; numerous vitamins, including C and E; and many minerals.

Protein Powders

I feel that protein powders, blended into shakes or smoothies, deserve a place in a good diet, mainly if you're active and work out regularly. Drinking a protein shake, for example, within forty-five to sixty minutes following a workout has been shown to create a hormonal environment in the body that supports muscle development. That's not hype, either, but scientifically validated knowledge we've known for a long time.

Although I prefer plant-based protein powders, you might want to try a product formulated with whey protein, casein protein, or both. Whey protein powder is a fast fuel because it is absorbed into your system quickly—and that's why it's effective as a post-workout supplement, especially when blended in a smoothie with a fast-fuel carb such as fruit.

Whey can also help alter body composition for the better. By that I mean more muscle and less body fat. In 2011, the *Journal of Nutrition* published the results of a study in which overweight adults who supplemented their regular diets with whey lost body fat and trimmed their waistlines over a twenty-three-week period.

Casein protein is more of a slow protein, digested slowly and absorbed slowly by the body. This slow-release attribute may help prevent a catabolic state (protein breakdown) by continually supplying amino acids to the body, particularly overnight. A casein-formulated protein powder is good for a bedtime snack to support recovery processes while you sleep, or as a snack during the day to supply your body with a steady stream of protein.

Again, I've steered more toward vegan protein powders, namely, brown rice or pea protein powders, in order to shift to a diet that includes more vegetables and fewer processed foods. Brown rice protein powder, derived from whole-grain rice, is around 90 percent protein and complete with all nine essential amino acids. It is well absorbed by the body, making it a great post-workout fuel. Pea protein is a slow-digesting protein, like casein. This means it may be able to keep you full longer than whey does, and it may also help you combat cravings more effectively. In fact, in a study published in 2011 in the *Nutrition Journal*, researchers discovered that subjects who drank pea protein powder smoothies *before* a meal ate significantly fewer calories at the meal than subjects who drank whey protein smoothies before eating. Pea protein might just be a great natural appetite suppressant. See my recipes starting on page 121 for ideas on how to incorporate pea protein and other protein powders into some delicious smoothies.

Regardless of what type of protein powder you use, choose a "weight gainer" product if you're trying to bulk up and put on a lot of mass. In the smoothie section, I've added a couple of high-calorie shakes. These can be used if one of your main physique goals is to gain muscle. The best time to use these high-calorie shakes is within forty-five minutes after your workout.

Creatine

I'm a fan of the supplement creatine monohydrate because it has been so well tested.

Creatine increases your supply of ATP, a compound that supplies energy to the body. The more creatine your muscles have, the more ATP they can produce and the longer you can exercise. Several studies have found that creatine augments strength and muscle gains when used in conjunction with regular strength-training workouts.

Available as a powder, creatine can be easily mixed into smoothies or protein shakes. You can even dissolve it in tea. Take 2 to 5 grams (usually a scoop or two) before and after workouts.

One caution here: if you supplement with creatine, be sure to drink ample water daily—at least eight to ten glasses. That's because when creatine is shunted into your muscles, it tends to drag water in with it. You've got to keep plenty of water circulating in and out of your system when supplementing with creatine, or else you may put an unnecessary burden on your kidneys.

SUPPLEMENT TIMING

I'm not a stickler when it comes to advice on when to take your supplements. Take them whenever it's convenient! Other than that, here's how the Body Fuel plan might incorporate supplements.

Meal 1: Body Fuel breakfast, including homemade juice supplemented with green powder

Meal 2: post-workout protein shake with fruit and creatine

Meal 3: Body Fuel lunch

Meal 4: protein shake

Meal 5: Body Fuel dinner

Meal 6 (optional): protein shake made with slow-digesting casein or pea protein

THE FINAL WORD

- Get your doctor's advice before adding any supplement to your diet, and take it only if medically approved—unless it's a protein powder, protein bar, or a greens supplement (these are actually food).
- Consult your doctor regarding any nutrient deficiencies you might have that can be corrected by supplementation.
- Stay on high alert when it comes to supplement hype.
- Don't try to replace a healthful diet with a bunch of supplements. Fresh, colorful fruits and vegetables and natural whole grains provide a nutritional edge that can't be duplicated by pills, tablets, and capsules.

PART 4

THE BODY FUEL WORKOUT

CHAPTER 11

A QUICKER SYSTEM FOR FASTER RESULTS

Drop and give me ten . . . ten minutes, that is.

If you've had a tough time making exercise a habit or squeezing it into an already crowded schedule, I've got some terrific news for you: muscle toning, strength, and fitness can be achieved in ten minutes several times a week, and you don't even have to join a gym or travel across town to an exercise class.

Welcome to the Body Fuel workout. It's a short but vigorous workout program that uses body-weight exercises to help you lose fat, rev up your metabolism, and build strength.

Body-weight exercises do not require dumbbells, barbells, resistance bands, stability balls, or clunky machines—only your own body as your gym equipment. Your weight provides the resistance that leads to greater strength and definition.

Body-weight exercises can build more muscle than weightlifting because they activate many muscles at once. This factor ramps up your metabolism and sculpts muscles better than isolation-type exercises, the kind you do using gym equipment. Also, body-weight moves can burn more fat than aerobics and are safer than most workouts, since these exercises also develop balance and stability, helping to prevent injuries. And keep this in mind: body-weight exercises can be done in your living room, hotel room, backyard, or office.

Now don't waltz off and think body-weight exercises are wimpy. Consider this: if you've ever done squats, push-ups, or challenging yoga-type moves, you know that these really work your muscles hard. And it makes sense. Movements that require strength, endurance, balance, flexibility, and coordination are harder than exercises that require only one of these skills. To prove my point at the highest levels, take a look at the physiques of Olympic gymnasts.

Body-weight movements have been at the core of strength and conditioning programs for the most elite fighting forces in the military (think really tough guys) for literally thousands of years. Typically, they're used either exclusively or along with other training methods when soldiers are deployed or while preparing for a deployment.

In 1997 as a Special Operations recruit, I was introduced to an elite (and grueling!) strength and conditioning program that relied primarily on body-weight exercises. Our first ten weeks of training were to test our mettle, and there was a high drop-out rate. Granted, most of that attrition was due to water training, but a lot of it was influenced by countless hours of body-weight exercises. I remember the time when a thousand nonstop team push-ups were doled out on a Friday afternoon to "punish" the team for a few of us using too much athletic tape to strengthen our extremely flimsy snorkels! Admittedly, we had been warned the day before to remove it.

Regardless of how body-weight workouts were used, I noticed massive changes in my own physique and the physiques of others. I got hooked on this form of training and have been using it ever since to develop both mental and physical qualities in people I train.

I don't mean to give you the impression that military-inspired workouts are too hard-core. Not at all. Body-weight exercises can be adjusted to match any fitness level. Even the standard push-up can start out as a very basic move. You can begin with your hands elevated on a wall or countertop. As you get stronger, find lower and lower surfaces to place your hands on, until you can do the movement with your hands and feet on the ground. Then you can elevate your feet to make it still harder. And if that becomes too easy, try going through that entire progression using one-armed push-ups. Also, you can pause for one or two seconds at the top or bottom of a movement to increase the intensity. Challenge your stability, balance, and coordination by performing movements on unstable surfaces. Push-ups can be done with your hands on a ball, for example. You can also boost benefits by exerting greater control over movements—lower your body weight slowly and lift it as fast as you can. Increased control with body-weight exercises leads to increased control in day-to-day life. And that's just a push-up.

So are machines a thing of the past?

I believe there's a place for everything, but there's nothing magical about a barbell or any weight-training apparatus for that matter. If you did three sets of twelve repetitions of push-ups to the point of failure (where your muscles give out and you can't do any more), that's the same load on your muscles as doing three sets of twelve repetitions to the point of failure on the bench press. Actually, with the push-up, the supporting musculature is much more involved. The key lies in knowing which exercise variations to use in order to stay within the appropriate rep range. The same principle also applies to pulling, squatting, hip hinging, and core-strengthening movements.

YOU ARE YOUR OWN GYM: THE BENEFITS OF BODY-WEIGHT WORKOUTS

There are so many other benefits to using your body as your own gym, but probably the biggest benefit is that it's time-efficient. You can work out anywhere and anytime. Let's say you're at your desk, slumped over your computer and feeling draggy. All you have to do is get up and pound out about ten minutes of body-weight moves. Afterward, you'll feel reenergized for the rest of the day. Plus, you'll wake up refreshed and ready for anything the next day. You could also get up from your desk every fifteen minutes to do a few reps with any of my exercises. Throughout an entire workday, that's a lot of exercise!

The number one excuse why people don't exercise is time, but with body-weight exercise that's not the case. There really isn't an excuse for it because the routines take only ten minutes. Who can't find ten minutes?

Plus, you don't have to worry about doing any extra aerobics (unless you want to). The Body Fuel workout allows more of a cardiovascular component because you can move rapidly from one exercise to the next and you're using many muscles at once. This elevates your heart rate steadily, so you achieve a built-in aerobic effect.

Body-weight exercises also improve sports performance because they tend to be functional. That is, they don't just make you good at exercising; you'll develop effective ways of moving that will improve your performance in day-to-day life and in sports. Rather than becoming proficient at using machines or lifting barbells, you'll become proficient at moving your body through all planes of motion—up/down, forward/backward, laterally, and rotating—a sharp contrast to traditional weight training, which uses only a single plane of motion. My workouts maximally strengthen the ways we move naturally with the smallest possible sacrifice of time. Your ability to squat, lunge, push, pull, and rotate while maintaining ideal joint alignment will be drastically improved, and you'll see added strength, endurance, speed, power, balance, flexibility, and coordination. Simply put, you become much better at using your body.

If you already do some exercising, you may feel that you've hit a plateau or that your workouts have become boring. If so, then body-weight exercises may give you more options when access to a gym is unavailable, time is limited, or you want to kick up your current routine.

Hoo-ya!

Benefits of Body-Weight Exercises and an Active Lifestyle

- Weight loss and long-term weight control
- Favorable improvements in body composition (more muscle, less body fat)
- Greater physical strength

- Prevention of life-threatening diseases, such as cardiovascular disease, diabetes, and cancer
- Reduction and control of high blood pressure
- Better bone strength and health
- Improved mental focus
- Stress relief and management
- Possible prevention of injuries
- Improved self-confidence and self-image
- Development of good posture
- Enhanced athletic skills and abilities
- Development of coordination and balance
- Improved flexibility

THE BODY FUEL DIET + THE BODY FUEL WORKOUT

You're also going to achieve far better weight loss results when you do the Body Fuel workout along with the diet explained in Part 1. Exercise is a huge part of any lose-fat, build-muscle program. You won't get the results without combining the two.

If you try to lose weight without exercising, you'll drop pounds, but you'll likely also lose some valuable calorie-burning muscle. Body fat will come off faster if you do body-weight workouts while cycling your calories, instead of dieting without exercise. Body-weight exercises help speed up your metabolism and cause you to burn calories faster—benefits that last several hours after you've stopped exercising. Research affirms this: the more muscle you activate in a workout, the higher your metabolism stays for the next twenty-four to forty-eight hours. That means your body keeps burning fat long after your workout is over, even while you're sleeping.

Maintaining your lean muscle tissue with exercise is the best way to sustain a high-calorie-burning metabolism. This will help you keep the weight off in the long run and helps ensure that it won't return or be a persistent problem.

Use the Body Fuel workouts to build the entire spectrum of fitness—strength, endurance, balance, coordination, and so forth—with the smallest possible sacrifice of time. Body-weight training, plus a healthful diet, is the straightest line between where you are now and where you want to be.

In the next chapter, I'll introduce you to some moves that will help you get sleeker, stronger, and richer (no expensive gym membership or equipment required)—and the only price is a little sweat.

MY SIX SUCCESS PRINCIPLES

1. *Consistency.* Truly the number one success ingredient. Whether you want to lose fat, gain muscle, or some combination of the two, consistency in nutrition and training is king. This means sticking to the diet plan every day and always working out at least three times per week. This may sound obsessive to you, but I believe taking care of your well-being needs to be a priority, not just to change your physique but to ingrain positive habits that will ensure success in all the other areas of your life. Nothing will ever work unless you keep showing up, week after week, with no slacking off. With body-weight exercises, this couldn't be easier.

2. *Recovery.* Allow yourself some generous downtime between workouts. These rest periods are referred to as "recovery time." Many people get so gung ho that they work out every day. Ironically, this habit can lead to inadequate or slow results (overtraining). Muscles grow, develop, and tone up *between* workouts, not during them. For most people with full-time jobs and family priorities, three or four 10-to-20-minute, non-consecutive body-weight workouts a week is the perfect place to start.

3. *Regularity.* The body does not respond for long to workouts that are an unplanned, disorganized mishmash; rather, it thrives on regularity and routine. As my air traffic controller instructor used to say, "We need a system and then a plan—that's when we're dangerous." Or to paraphrase: that's when we get in

super shape. It's best to set goals and regularly and methodically do the exercises that get us there the fastest.

4. *Variety.* Variety is the spice of life, but when it comes to exercise, it doesn't mean performing a different exercise every time you work out. You can certainly do the same exercises year after year. But whether your body responds to those exercises depends on how much you vary your volume and your intensity. If you don't pump up the volume or increase your intensity, your body will have no reason to continue changing.

5. *Overload.* To activate increases in strength, mass, and tone, you must subject a muscle to an overload. This means putting your muscles under stress that they are unaccustomed to. The body constantly requires new stimulus to force it to change for the better. There are several ways to achieve overload with body-weight training:

    - *Perform a greater number of repetitions or sets with the same exercise each workout.*
    - *Reduce the length of rest periods between sets.*
    - *Perform some even harder exercises (to learn some, go to MarkLauren.com).*
    - *Increase the speed with which you perform exercises.*
    - *Use a combination of the above methods to increase the degree of overload you place on each muscle group.*

6. *Progression.* Start where you are, be patient, and gradually increase training volume and intensity. More isn't better. Just enough is enough. Always look to advance the difficulty of your workouts without overloading yourself too much. The more you progress, the more you'll see it in your body. To get to the advanced stage, try additional body-weight exercises, do harder variations of each, perform more sets and reps, rest less between sets, speed up your tempo,

or do any combination of these. But be aware that it's also possible for a program to progress too rapidly, causing overtraining.

Getting a great body doesn't happen overnight. It's not something you do every now and then and be done with. It's about staying dedicated to a healthful lifestyle that includes exercise and proper nutrition. Every couple of months, reevaluate your program. What's working? What isn't working? What can you do better? Ask and answer these questions, then make the necessary course corrections, whether that means adding in a few different exercises or switching to a higher intensity. If you don't keep yourself challenged, your progress will stall and you'll likely lose interest. Keep moving forward. Stay the course, and you'll see significant gains in your shape and health. Nothing is more motivating than progress!

To get started, read through the exercise descriptions and study the illustrated examples of how to perform them. You don't need a personal trainer. Let the pictures of me and the exercise instructions be your guide. After a few workouts, you won't even need to consult this chapter. You'll have all the moves memorized.

HOW IT WORKS

Follow the exercises in the order given, including the warm-up exercises at the beginning and the cool-down exercises at the end. You'll find three easy-to-follow workouts after the exercise descriptions.

WHAT YOU'LL NEED

Not a thing! That's the beauty of using your body as your own gym. (Of course, get some comfortable workout attire and make some space in which to move around.)

Ready to get started? Let's go!

CHAPTER 12

ON YOUR MARK, GET SET . . . GO! THE BODY FUEL EXERCISES

THE WARM-UP EXERCISES

Dirty Dogs

STARTING POSITION

Begin with your hands and knees on the floor. Keep your knees together.

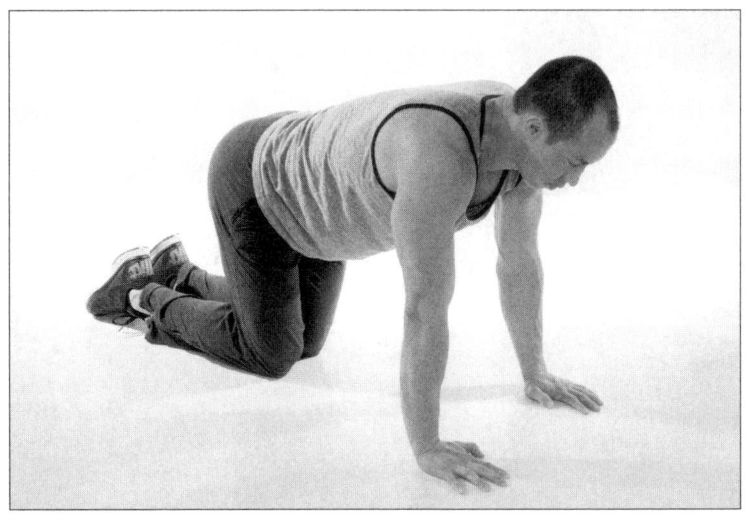

ACTION

Keeping your right knee bent at a 90-degree angle, lift it as high as you can. Briefly hold the top position, squeezing your right glute. Lower your right leg to complete the repetition. Perform 10 repetitions on the right. Switch sides and perform 10 repetitions on the left.

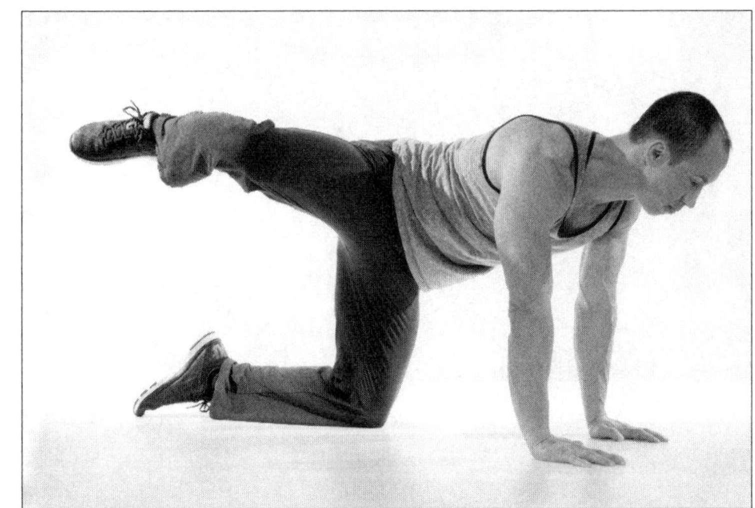

Side Lying T-Spine Rotation

STARTING POSITION

Lie on your right side with your knees tucked so that there is a 90-degree bend at the knees and hips. Your arms should be extended in front of you with your left hand placed on top of your right hand.

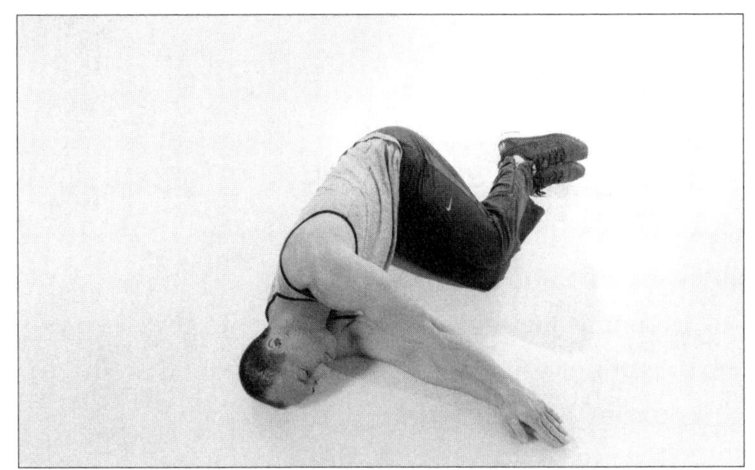

ACTION

Raise your left arm straight up and then lower it to the opposite side of your torso. Get your left shoulder blade and arm as close to the ground as possible. Return to the starting position. Do 10 repetitions on your right. Switch sides and perform 10 repetitions on your left.

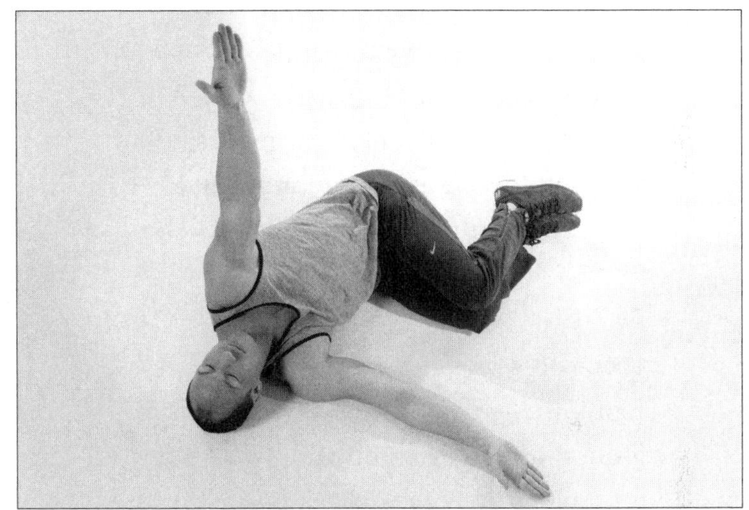

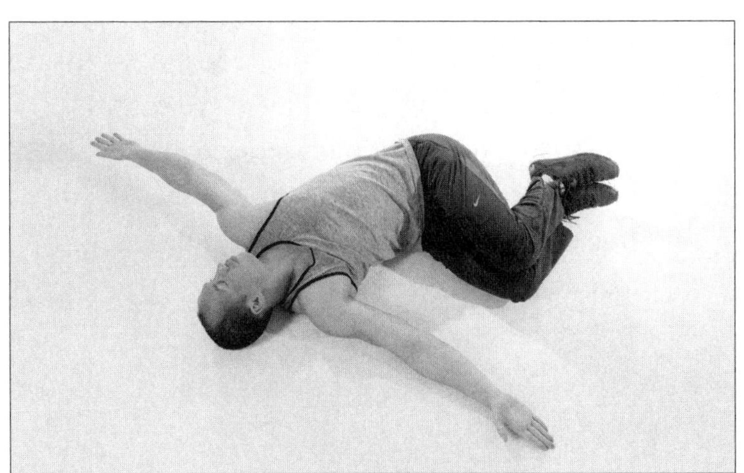

Isometric Saxon Lunge

STARTING POSITION

Lunge forward on your right leg to get into the bottom of a lunge. Extend your arms overhead. Your elbows should be straight with your hands placed on top of one another as if you're about to dive into a pool. Your right knee should be directly over the top of your right ankle. The toes of your left foot should be pointing away from your body.

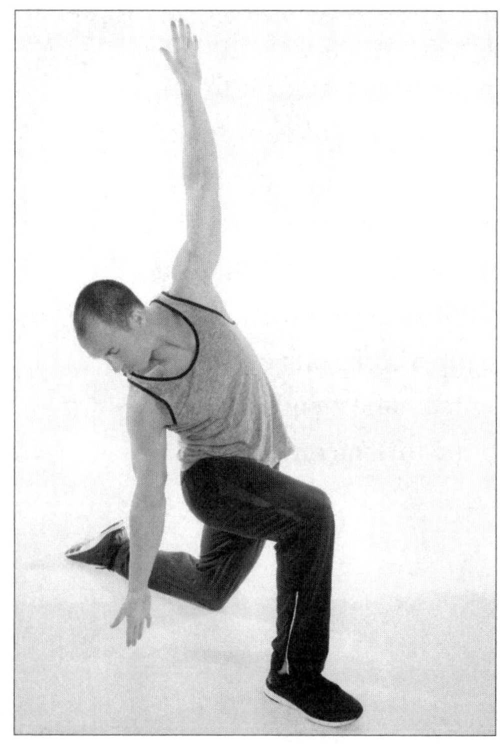

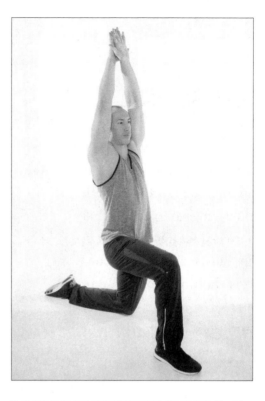

ACTION

From this position, press your left foot into the ground, and flex your left glute muscle. Reach down toward the ground with your right hand while reaching up toward the ceiling with your left hand. You should feel a stretch along the left side of your body. Hold this position for 5 seconds before returning to the starting position. Do 5 repetitions. Switch sides and do 5 more repetitions.

Zombie Squats

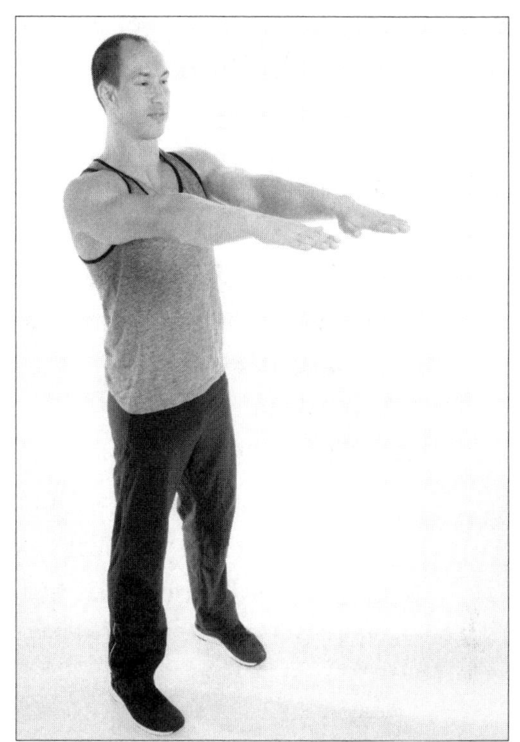

STARTING POSITION

Stand upright with your feet about shoulder-width apart and your chest slightly elevated. Extend your arms out in front of your body like a zombie. Your toes should be pointing straight ahead, not out to the sides.

ACTION

Push your hips back. Bend your knees and sink your hips down as deeply as you can while keeping your back from being fully rounded. Avoid letting your knees turn in toward each other. If you're flexible, you'll be able to sink all the way down until your hips are resting on your calves. Once you cannot go any deeper without putting your back into full flexion, reverse the motion, squeeze your glutes, and stand upright again. Perform 15 repetitions.

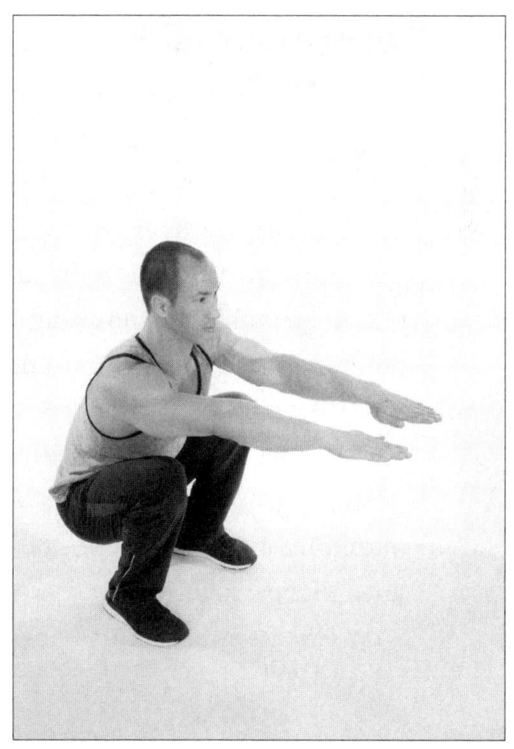

MAIN EXERCISES

Streamline Back Lunges

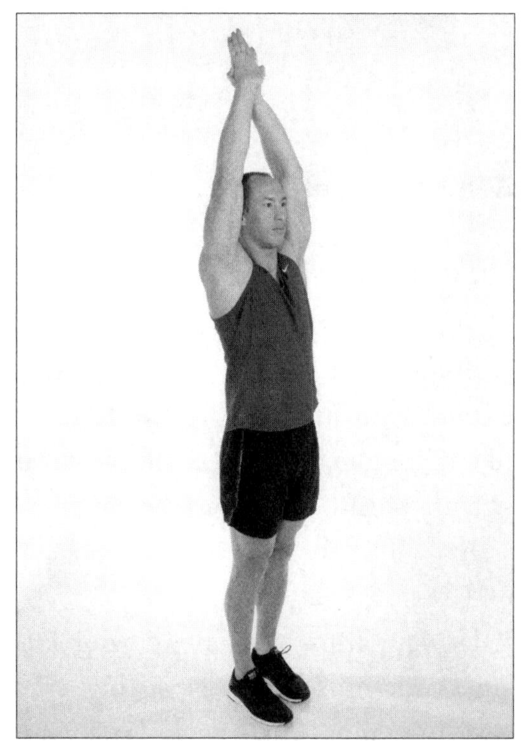

TARGETED MUSCLES

Legs, glutes, spinal erectors of the back, and core

STARTING POSITION

Stand tall and upright with your feet close together and your arms extended overhead as if you're about to jump into a pool.

ACTION

Take a big step backward with your right leg. Bend your left knee and sink your hips back and down until your right knee almost touches the ground. Step far enough back so that your left knee is directly over the top of your left ankle. With your right knee just off the ground and pointing straight down, reverse the motion and stand upright again.

Repeat the exercise with the opposite leg. Throughout this exercise maintain a tall, upright torso with your biceps covering your ears. Keep your elbows as straight as possible.

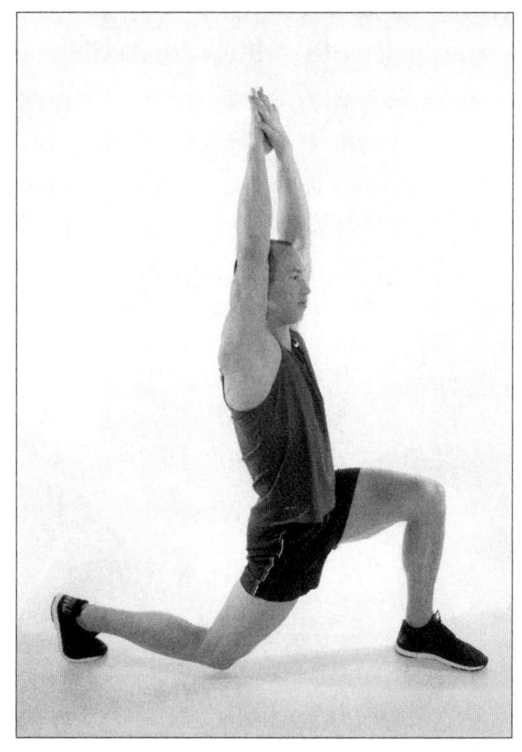

Bodyrocks

TARGETED MUSCLES

Core, shoulders, latissimus dorsi of the back, and quadriceps (front thighs)

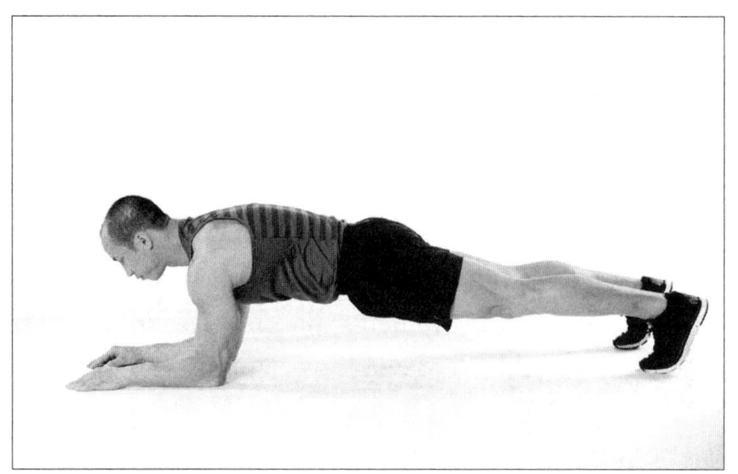

STARTING POSITION

Place your body in the starting position of a push-up with your body straight from head to heels. Lower yourself down onto your forearms. Your elbows should be directly underneath your shoulders.

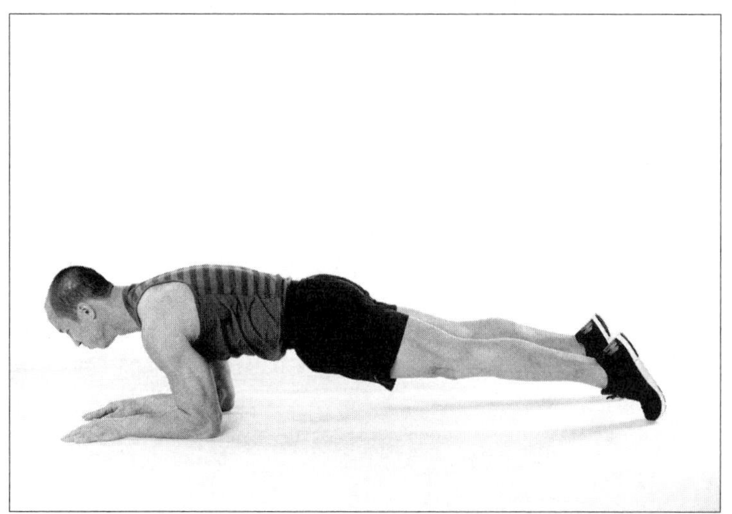

ACTION

From this position, rock your body back and forth. Go forward and backward as far as you can without lifting or lowering your hips. Continue rocking back and forth while maintaining a straight line from head to heels.

Squat Thrusts

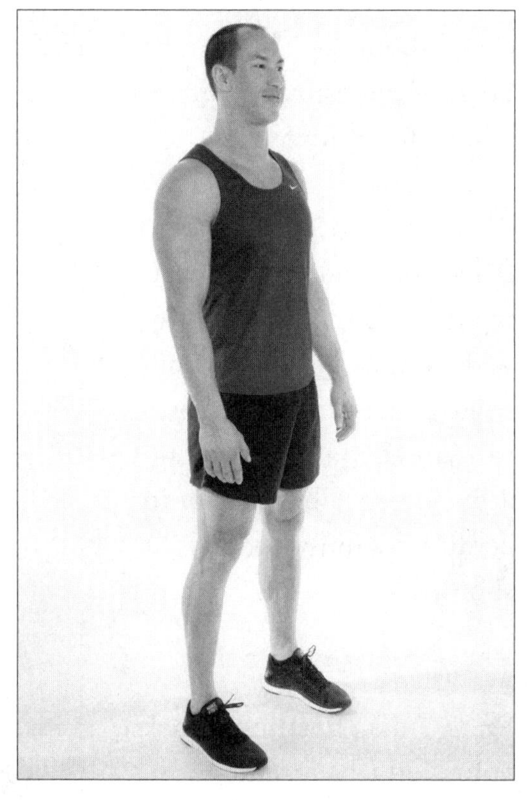

TARGETED MUSCLES

Legs, core, shoulders, triceps, and latissimus dorsi of the back

STARTING POSITION

Stand with your feet shoulder-width apart and your arms at your side. Push your hips back, bend the knees, and place your hands on the ground.

ACTION

Jump your feet back so that you land in the starting position of a push-up. Your hands should be underneath your shoulders and your body should be straight from head to heels with your abdominals drawn in and tightened. Jump your feet back up toward your hands. Then stand upright, returning to the starting position.

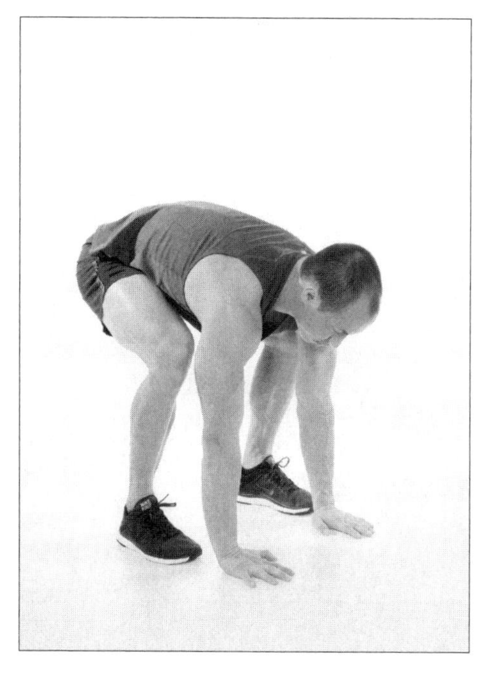

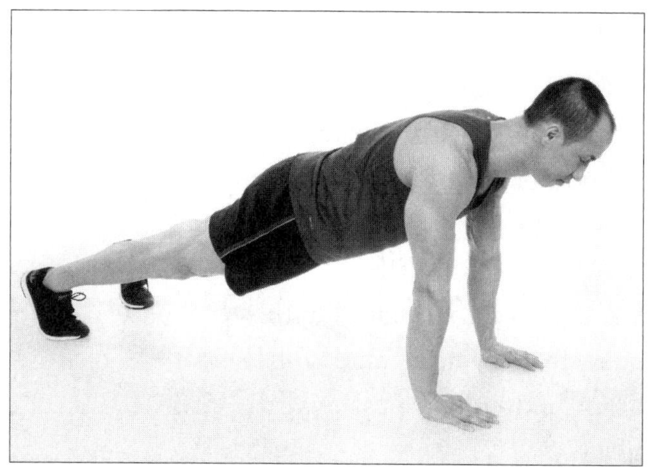

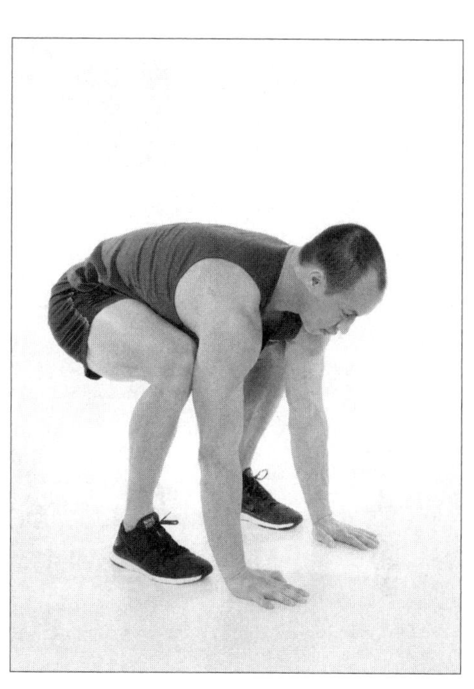

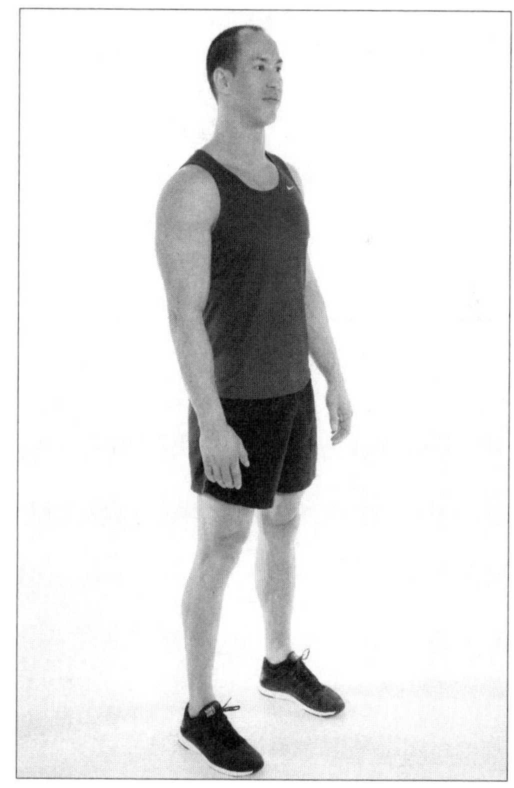

Arm Haulers

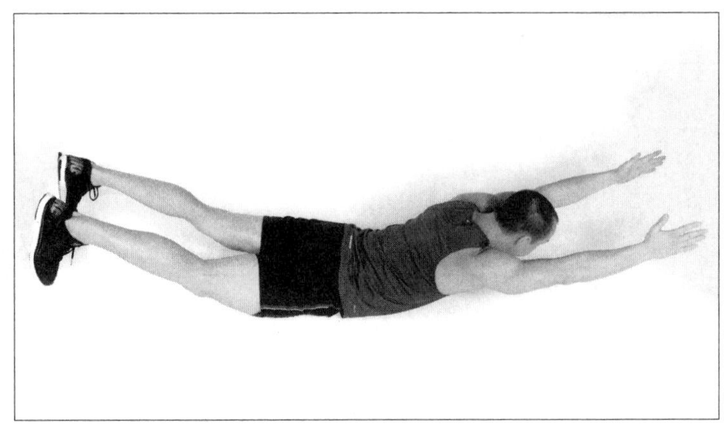

TARGETED MUSCLES

Spinal erectors of the back, shoulders, and trapezius

STARTING POSITION

Lie on your stomach with your feet together and your arms extended past your head.

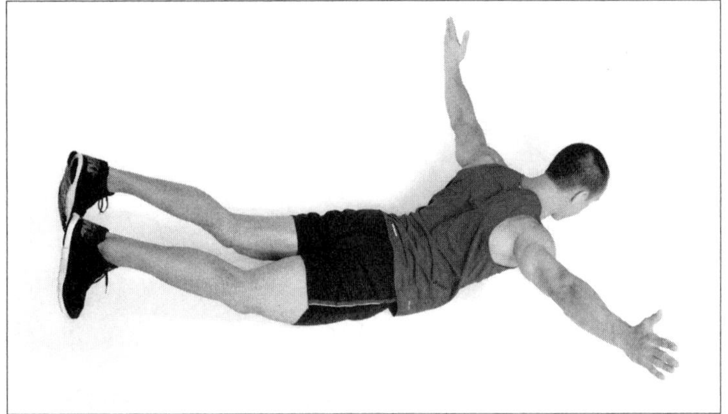

ACTION

Lift your arms and legs off the ground. While keeping your limbs elevated, bring your arms to the sides of your body. Return your arms back to the starting position and repeat. Throughout this movement, your thumbs should point up toward the sky.

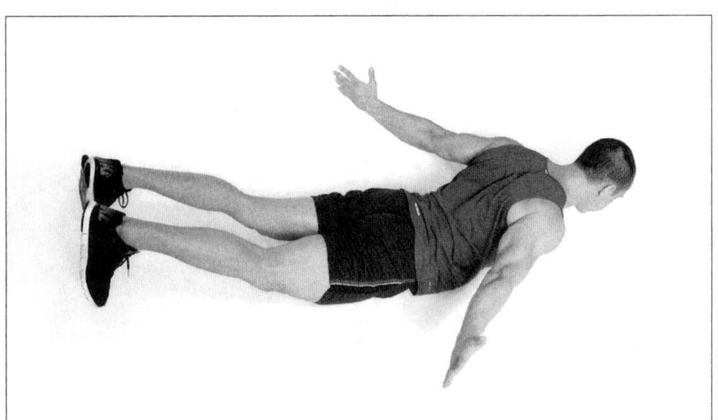

COOL-DOWN STRETCHES

Straddle Reach

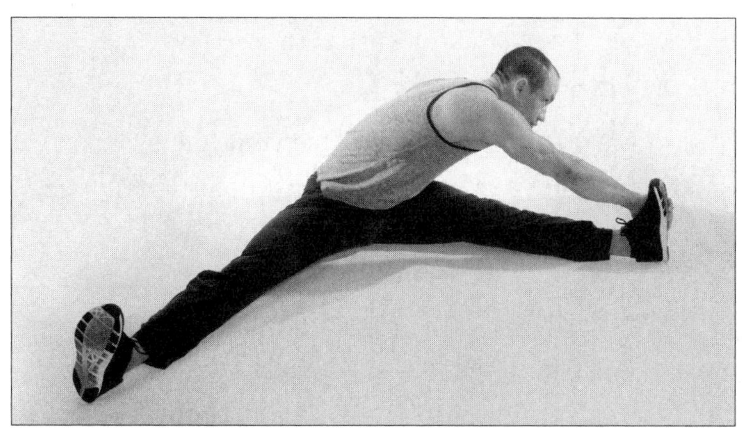

STARTING POSITION

Sit on the floor with your legs spread far enough apart that you feel a light stretch in your groin. Sit up straight, with your toes pulled back and pointing up at the ceiling.

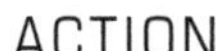

ACTION

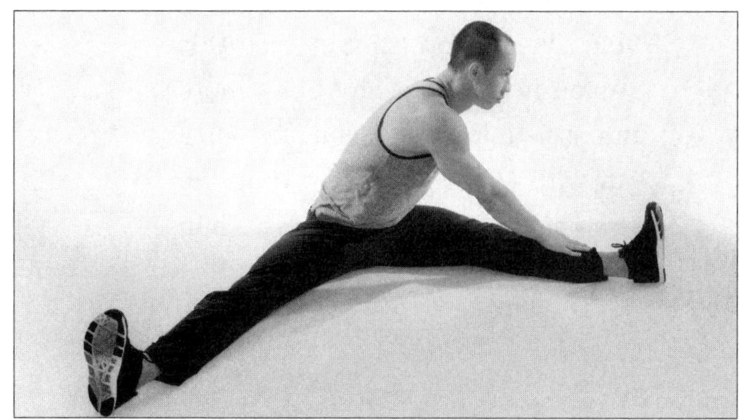

With your right hand, reach as far to the outside of your left foot as you can. Hold this stretch for about 20–30 seconds before switching sides. If you can't reach your foot, reach to the outside of your shins or knees. Avoid fully rounding your back during this stretch.

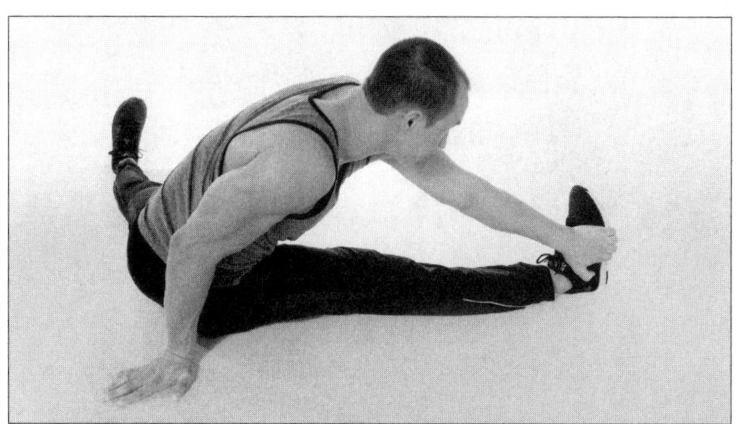

Figure 4 Hip Stretch

STARTING POSITION

Lie on your back and place your left foot on your right thigh, just below the knee.

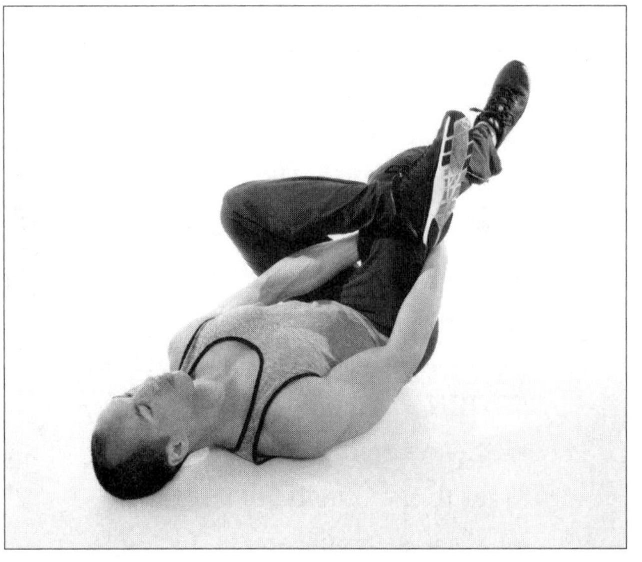

ACTION

With both hands, grab your right thigh underneath your left foot and pull your right leg in toward your chest. You should feel this stretch in your left hip. For a more intense stretch, push your left knee out with your right elbow. Hold the stretch for 20–30 seconds. Then switch sides and repeat.

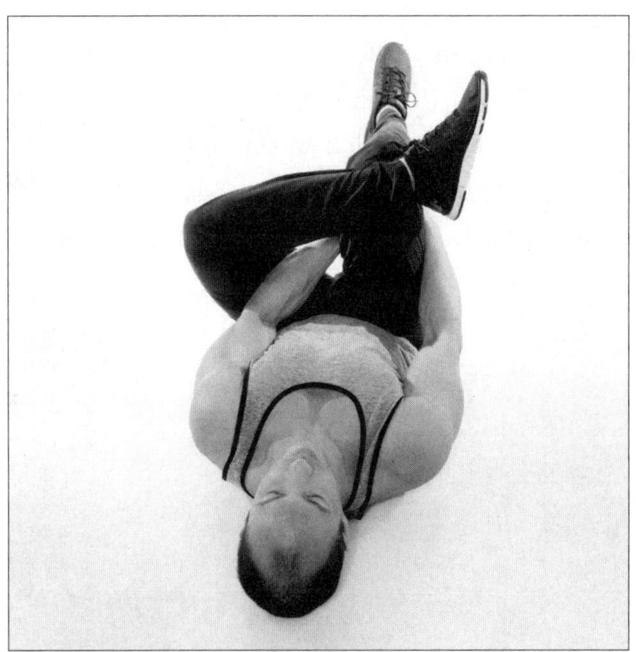

Scorpion Twist

STARTING POSITION

Lie on your stomach with your feet together, your left arm extended past your head, and your right arm perpendicular to your body. Bend your right arm so that there is a 90-degree bend at the elbow.

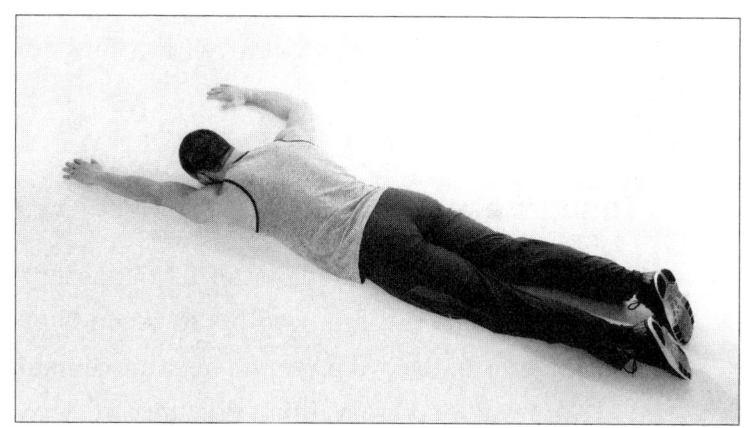

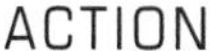

ACTION

Bend your left knee and lift it straight up. Now twist so that your left foot ends up as far on the right side of your body as possible. While twisting, keep your left armpit as close to the ground as possible. This stretch lengthens the lats, pecs, and hip flexors while improving rotation. Hold this position for 20–30 seconds. Repeat on the opposite side.

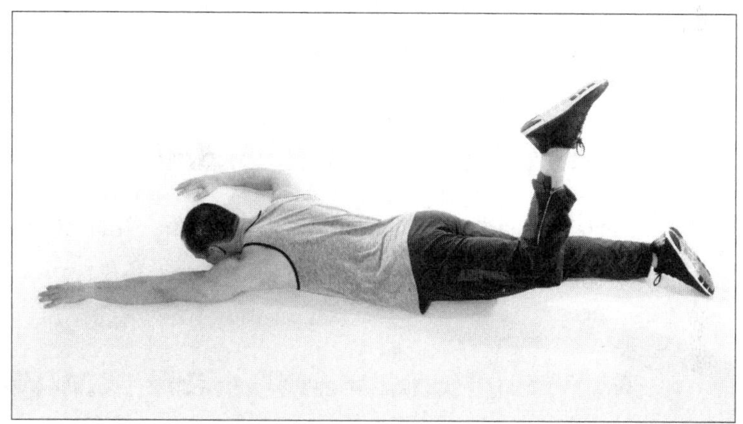

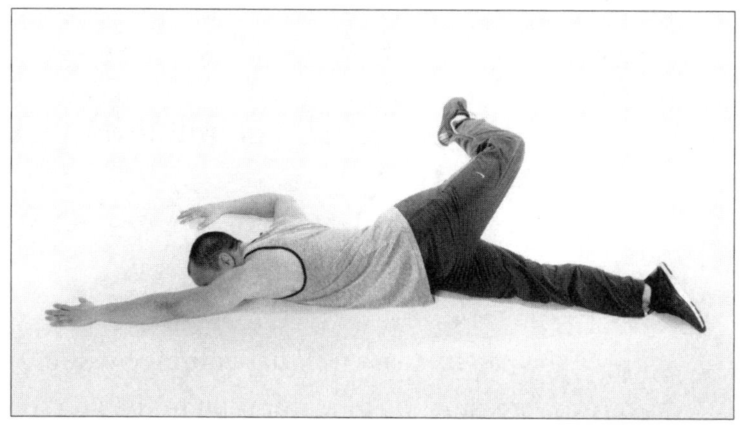

WORKOUTS

You can use any of these workouts exclusively or in conjunction with one another. After completing the warm-up as prescribed above, perform one of the below workouts. Then unwind with a few minutes of stretching for the cool-down.

Timed Sets (Monday)

Perform each of the exercises for 3–5 consecutive sets. Each set will consist of 30 seconds of work, followed by 30 seconds of rest. Once you've completed all sets for an exercise, go on to the next movement.

You can increase training intensity by decreasing the rest intervals, and you can increase training volume by performing more reps per set or by doing more sets for an exercise.

Circuit Training (Wednesday)

Perform each exercise for 40 seconds. Rest 20 seconds, then move on to the next exercise. Rotate through all exercises 3–5 times.

As Many Rounds as Possible (AMRAP, Friday)

Perform the below exercises, with the prescribed number of reps, for as many rounds as possible in ten minutes.

- Streamline Back Lunges—10 alternating reps (5 reps per leg)
- Bodyrocks—15 reps
- Squat Thrusts—10 reps
- Arm Haulers—15 reps

You can increase training volume by doing more rounds in the allotted time or by increasing the total duration of the workout, up to 20 minutes.

CHAPTER 13

BODY FUEL IN THE REAL WORLD

Whether you've already done a victory lap around the scale or are closing in on your weight loss and fitness goals, plant the thought in your head that what you're doing has no beginning and no end. The Body Fuel plan is something that's now a part of your life, not just a diet. It's a lifestyle change.

I know you can make and sustain that change. This plan is livable—indefinitely—and livable is the opposite of yo-yo. You can do this the rest of your life.

To increase your chances of making that happen, what else should you be doing? What helps is knowing how to navigate the obstacle course of lifelong nutrition and health, from dining out to traveling to preventing weight gain.

FUELING UP AT RESTAURANTS

I don't know about you, but I'm not going to stay home and chew on celery. I love eating out at restaurants too much to give it up. I like the food, some wine on occasion, and the social aspect of being with friends and family.

On the Body Fuel plan, your dining-out paradigm doesn't have to drastically change. In fact, it's remarkably simple to eat out practically anywhere and stick to the plan. First, scout out the menu, looking for foods that are included on Body Fuel. The first question you ask yourself is: *What protein should I choose?* This could be a steak, grilled chicken, some fish, or other protein that won't be swimming in cream sauce.

Next: *What should my slow and fast fuels be?* You can order a salad with some oil and vinegar dressing on the side, a vegetable medley, or a fast-fuel carb such as rice, a baked potato, or a sweet potato. If you're doing Block 1, choose as many slow-fuel vegetables as you can. On Block 2 or 3, simply control how many fast-fuel carbs you order. Drink lots of water, too.

Have questions about the menu? Restaurant personnel usually are very willing to discuss the menu with you and accommodate your requests. Fortunately, restaurants are responding to the 75 percent of consumers who say they try to eat more healthfully while dining out, according to the National Restaurant Association.

I know that when I go to a restaurant, I'll be heading home with a second meal. That's simply because restaurant portions are as massive as the Canadian Rockies. Sometimes I'll ask for a doggie bag up front and put half the meal in it right away. I just took care of my lunch or dinner for the next day. This is a great time-saving, money-saving, waistline-saving tactic to use.

When dining out, I prefer to skip those all-you-can-eat places (too tempting) and chain restaurants, where the food isn't at all fresh since it's usually transported in from parts unknown. Instead, I focus on unique establishments, from mom-and-pop restaurants to little hole-in-the-wall places, that will provide me with local fare or food that's cooked fresh and from scratch. Southeast Asian and Japanese restaurants are also good bets, with their variety of vegetables and proteins.

Now about navigating cocktails. Alcohol tends to drive up cortisol levels in your body, and that's a bad deal. Cortisol seems to direct fat right to your waistline. (This is probably why so many beer-guzzling men have beer guts, but the same unflattering profile can happen to women, too.)

Until you get to your weight goal, it's a good idea to forgo alcohol for consistent weight loss. After you've achieved your ideal weight, enjoy some alcohol in moderate amounts. Moderation typically means one drink daily for women and two drinks daily for men. One drink is 12 ounces of regular beer, 5 ounces of wine, or 1.5 ounces of distilled liquor. Or look to the weekends, when you dine out, to have a drink with your meal.

Drinking more than that on a frequent basis can be risky. The reason is that alcohol, besides its fat-promoting side effects, jeopardizes your body's use of vitamins and minerals, including thiamin, vitamin B_6, and calcium. Furthermore, chronic alcohol abuse has negative side effects on every organ in the body, particularly the liver. Drinking alcohol in large amounts can also lead to accidents, as well as social, psychological, and emotional problems.

Hoo-ya!

How to Have a Healthful Meal at a Drive-Through

Yes, you can get a decent meal at a fast-food joint, though I'm not a big fan of these places. My overall advice is to eat at a fast-food restaurant only if it's your sole option.

Fast-food menus are always changing, so let me give you some general guidelines on how to order.

Burger joints. Order a burger and don't eat the bun unless you need your fast-fuel for the day. Have a salad to round out the meal, and select a low-calorie salad dressing. A veggie burger or a grilled chicken sandwich isn't a bad choice, either; they're usually low in calories. Hold the mayo on any sandwich and have some mustard instead. Avoid items such as crispy chicken sandwiches, bacon cheeseburgers (or any cheeseburgers, for that matter), and fried fish anything.

Sub shops. Order salads and/or vegetable soups that are not cream-based. A six-inch veggie sub is a healthful choice if you need a fast-fuel. Again, no mayo; go the mustard route.

Fried chicken establishments. Enter with caution! The wafting smell of fried chicken might be too seductive. But resistance is not futile. Select a roasted chicken entrée with a side of green beans or corn, and get out of there as fast as you can!

Mexican fast food. Here your best bets are chicken or beef strips served in flour tortillas. Skip fatty items such as nachos, enchiladas, burritos, and so forth. Oh, and about those taco salads: they're loaded with calories (sometimes up to 900) and fat. Pass them by.

Asian fast food. I've found that you can pick up a decent meal at one of these fast-food restaurants. Usually they offer some type of chicken that isn't breaded or fried but still tastes good. Plate it up with a double order of steamed vegetables, and you've got a pretty nice Body Fuel meal.

FUELING UP ON THE ROAD

I live on the road for six months out of the year and have been doing so ever since I left my mother's home at age eighteen. I know something about how to stick to a healthful nutritional regime and maintain control over my meals when away from home, whether for business, on vacation, or just passing through.

I usually have a pretty healthful diet when I travel. I eat very clean, consuming mostly chicken and fish, vegetables, and fruit. Basically, whether I'm home or traveling, I look at food as fuel and energy to keep me going.

Often I'll swing by a local grocery store and buy travel staples such as canned tuna, boiled eggs, precut veggies, and fresh fruit, provided my accommodations have a mini-fridge. I love trail mix, too; it makes a great on-the-road fuel. And I drink lots of water.

One of the biggest travel challenges is fueling up at airports and on planes. Most foods found in airports are high in sugar, fat, and sodium and relatively low in nutrients. Plus, sitting in a confined airplane seat for a long time can cause fluid retention and swelling. I try to eat a healthful meal before I get to the airport, and I pack things like sliced apples, peeled oranges, trail mix, raw veggies, and grilled chicken to eat between meals so I'm not ravenously hungry by the time I make it to my destination. If I've planned poorly or encounter unexpected situations, I'll eat some fast food at the airport, making healthier, lighter choices whenever possible and eating just enough to prevent hunger.

BE YOUR OWN GYM WHILE TRAVELING

A related issue is exercising while on the road. This is really super simple with body-weight exercises, which can be done anywhere, including your hotel room. I don't need to go out and hunt for a gym, since my body is my own gym. Plus I travel a lot in places where the heat, traffic, and air quality aren't the best for outdoor exercise. But most important, training in my hotel room is fast, convenient, and highly effective.

My typical workout on the road includes a wide variety of push-ups, squats, lunges, and other body-weight exercises performed in fifteen-to-thirty-minute spurts of activity. I get a great aerobic and strength workout right in the privacy of my hotel. There are times, though, when I'm just too busy to set aside the time for a full workout. If you find yourself in a similar boat—exhausted and rushed—it's important to give yourself some options. One solution that works extremely well for me, both on the road and at home, is to take frequent exercise breaks throughout the day, especially if I'm sitting behind a computer. A variety of light sets of any exercise every fifteen to thirty minutes adds up to a good amount of work over the course of the day. You don't need to break a sweat, but each exercise break will keep your blood flowing and your mind active.

Get creative with your activity. If you're between connections or waiting in the airport, walk through the terminals.

It's important to stay consistently active while at home and while traveling. Remember that one of my principles for success is consistency. With body-weight exercises you can always work out *right now.* It doesn't need to be high intensity; it just needs to be consistent. Find a way.

SURVIVING THE HOLIDAYS

I'm going on the record to announce that I love holidays because of all the food around me. A major fitness magazine once asked me which foods I consider off-limits during the holidays. My answer was "None!"

Okay, you've probably heard that the average weight gain over the holidays is five to ten pounds. It can creep on, for sure, and I think we all know we're going to have lapses during holidays. That happens to everybody. Just keep it in perspective. Maybe you've overindulged, but don't get upset. Lapses here and there don't make you a failure.

You can prevent big problems, however, if you change your focus from dieting to healthful living during the holidays. First, a realistic goal is not to gain weight over the holidays; try to stay steady with your weight. Second, eat whatever you want—yes, you read that correctly! Just practice good portion control and stay active. Do whatever it takes to move your body. Practice your body-weight exercises. Walk your dog more, play in the yard with the kids after dinner, or throw the football around with your family members.

Often holidays are stressful with family members around. My advice: sweat it out. Exercise is one of the most effective ways to relieve emotional stress. It speeds up the production of natural feel-good chemicals called endorphins, plus it dissipates the buildup of cortisol in your body. Exercise also relieves muscular tension brought on by anxiety.

As long as you stay fairly active, you have my permission to indulge in all your favorite treats.

FUELING UP WITH YOUR FAMILY AND FRIENDS

What if you're on Block 1 or 2, restricting carbs, and your spouse wants pasta every night? Or your best friend insists on beer and pizza after work a few times a week?

There's no denying that these are tough issues, and your plans to get in shape will go more smoothly if you get your friends and family on board. They can be an enormous help to you if you recruit them to your side.

One of the best ways to do that is simply to keep in mind that where your health is involved, you come first. It's what you want that matters. That may sound a little selfish, but this is your life and your body. Your ability to serve others depends largely on how well you are able to care for yourself. Show people that you're committed to your priorities, stick to them, and before long you'll get converts. Your friends and family will see how great you feel, and this will give them the impetus to change, too. But you have to make a decision and commit.

It also helps if you communicate to people in your life that you need their support. Explain to them the premise of the Body Fuel plan. Go as far as to share with them your copy of this book. They need to know, especially if they've seen you fall off the diet wagon before, that this plan is different. Ask them to help you out by not offering you fattening foods, belittling your program, or tempting you in other ways. Ask them to never offer you food or tease or criticize you for your efforts. Don't expect your family to change the way they eat overnight, or restrict foods they like, but you can ask for their help. You'll be gradually introducing them to some new recipes and ways of eating, and ultimately they'll benefit.

Plenty of people can also attest to the power of dieting with a friend, buddy, or other family member. There's even hard science that supports this strategy. In a Miriam Hospital/Brown Medical School study of 109 overweight people, those who teamed up with a pal or relative who was also a committed dieter dropped twice as much weight as those who went solo or whose buddies didn't lose.

Dieting partners can help each other stay on track and celebrate small successes they might otherwise shrug off, especially when you're both working hard to get in shape. Make sure your partner is committed, too, and will be there for you, no matter what. If your friend ends up bingeing on cookies, reassure her that she'll be okay—and then a few days later say, "Okay, girl, let's get back on it." Try to lift each other up and be each other's safety net. Holding each other accountable is invaluable. Share recipes, food prep strategies, and healthful choices at particular restaurants. Whatever has helped you will help your buddy.

You might consider setting up a friendly competition. I perform at my best when others are watching or when I'm competing. Make a deal or a bet that every time you cheat or go off the plan, you've got to wash your partner's car, clean her house, buy him a healthful gift, or do fifty squats. Or you could set up a kitty and whoever cheats must contribute a certain sum of money to the pot, while whoever sticks with it and reaches his or her goal wins the money. If you make it a game, it's fun, and a little friendly competition never hurt anyone.

As helpful as it is to diet together, it's equally helpful to have a workout partner. Teaming up for exercise has a bunch of benefits. In a MyFitnessPal poll of 2,220 users, 65 percent said doing so made exercise more fun, 50 percent said they got a better workout that way, and 55 percent said it made them more likely to show up. You can learn and practice my body-weight exercises together and get other friends involved to make it a class. These exercises lend themselves very well to a supportive group experience. You could even work out alone for yourself once, then a second time to support a friend having trouble sticking to it.

MAINTAINING YOUR BODY FUEL SHAPE

After you get the pounds off, then what? Maintenance is even more challenging than losing the pounds, because you have to keep doing it every day. What follows are some recommendations for little things you can do to stay in shape and maintain your fabulous new self.

Keep Track

I do believe that periodically jumping on a scale (no more than every other week) to see if you're gaining, maintaining, or losing can be a useful tool. Weigh yourself at the same time of day each time. Write the number down and display it in a prominent place (like on your refrigerator) so you can't avoid it. Successful maintainers realize that their weight will fluctuate up and down like the stock market, but they set a range that they stay within, with a top number they won't exceed. So have a "trigger" weight—a number on the scale you absolutely will not surpass. Maybe it's a five-pound ceiling above your ideal goal weight. If you go over that weight, you get right back on Block 1 in order to take you back down to your ideal weight. Start right away, say at your next meal. This type of self-monitoring is one of the best tools you can use to maintain your results.

Begin Your Day with a Healthful Meal

A study of successful losers in the National Weight Control Registry (that's more than ten thousand people who lost an average of sixty-six pounds and kept it off for at least six years) found that if these people ate a healthful morning meal, they were better able to control their food intake the rest of the day. In fact, 78 percent of people in the registry reported that they ate breakfast every day.

Another secret uncovered by the registry is that the longer people worked at maintenance, the easier it became. The message here: hang in there!

Stick with Protein

University of Arizona scientists figured out how a group of 111 women kept off an average of ten pounds for a year after they completed a four-month weight loss program. Their secret: eating substantial amounts of protein throughout the day. Remember, protein is more satiating than carbs or even fat. Keep your weight off by continuing to follow my Body Fuel protein recommendations.

Veg Out

Experts are unanimous: eat lots of fruit and slow-fuel veggies. Fruit and slow-fuel vegetables help you feel fuller, leaving less room for high-fat, high-sugar junk. That's because these foods are high in water and fiber, and therefore volume. Continue to follow my Body Fuel recommendations for fruits and vegetables. Eating foods that have a lot of volume will keep you feeling full.

Use Block 3 as Your Maintenance Template

Block 3, with its additional fast-fuel carbs, is the ideal maintenance diet. It fuels you for daily activity, helps build and maintain muscle from your workouts, and gives you plenty of healthful nutrition. If you're ready to slip some desserts or alcoholic beverages back in your menu, substitute these for any fast-fuel carb on

Block 3. But the key here is moderation: stick to the allowable portion sizes! If you find yourself gaining weight, cut back on the number of splurges to one or two, or follow Block 1 to get back on track.

Stay Active

Working out as a permanent part of your lifestyle is a must for maintenance. More than 90 percent of successful losers from the National Registry of Weight Control are active at least an hour each day. Many walk for exercise, along with doing other forms of exercise. Scheduling your exercise times on a calendar, in a day planner, or on your smartphone—just like you'd do with other activities and events—will help ensure that you work out. If you're less organized and you find yourself skipping workouts, practice light body-weight movements throughout the day whenever you think of it. It doesn't need to be an epic effort; just move a bit.

Finally, any program that you can't stick with for the rest of your life isn't worth doing, even for a single day. Body Fuel is a program you can do for the rest of your life. It will transform your body and your health—and carry you successfully into the future.

EPILOGUE

FUELING YOUR PASSION

This is the end of the book but the beginning of a new life of health and fitness for you. We've covered a lot of ground, and I sincerely hope I've given you enough information and guidance to carry you through. You don't have to remember all of it, just as long as you remember the basic principles of Body Fuel. They're designed to last you a lifetime.

Let's do a final review:

- Follow the principle of calorie cycling for the sake of your metabolism and continued progress. The three blocks, with their variations in calories and carbs, will help you stay on track.
- Recognize the differences between slow-fuel and fast-fuel carbs. The fewer fast-fuel carbs you eat, the faster you'll lose body fat. At the same time, use fast-fuel carbs strategically to boost your muscle development, training, and energy levels.

- Eat at least five meals a day—three main meals and two snacks.
- Each meal consists of a protein, a carbohydrate, and fat. You'll obtain most of the fat you need directly from the food you eat.
- Look for ways to eat more slow-fuel carbs, namely vegetables, whether in salads, in juices, as snacks, or as accompaniments to main meals.
- Have a protein and a carb shortly after workouts—my smoothies are appropriate here—in order to take advantage of the post-workout window of opportunity for muscle growth, repair, and fat burning.
- Choose supplements wisely, and remember that they never take the place of real food.
- If you find that you're gaining body fat, use Block 2 or Block 1 to get your weight back down.
- Maintain a workout program, with emphasis on body-weight exercises, three to five times weekly, so you can burn even more fat and put on attractive muscle.
- Strive to steadily increase the difficulty of your workouts.

MIND FUEL

As you fuel your body with quality food, I believe you must also fuel your mind—and do so with quality thoughts and beliefs. I call this "mind fuel." Understand that the mind, like your muscles, increases in power and strength the more you train and exercise it.

In working with elite military forces, I observed something interesting: they are intensely motivated to do what they do—in the field, while deployed, in training, and in their physical workouts. And it isn't about being shouted at; it's about a deep sense of passion for their work and their mission.

I trust that you're serious about the shape of your body, inside and out. That seriousness gives you the motivation to eat right and get active. Bringing passion to your Body Fuel experience can take you to a whole new level. Passion is critical mind fuel that nourishes your commitment with greater intensity, gives you the mental energy to confront excuses that block the pursuit of your goals, and builds your self-confidence and self-respect.

Let's dig a little deeper into the role of passion—and how you can develop and use it as mind fuel to improve performance and strengthen your motivation.

In developing your passion, continually ask yourself this key question: Why do you want to eat right and get in shape? It may be to look great, to fit into a smaller size, for quality of life, to prevent disease, to have more energy, to sharpen your mind, or all of the above.

To reinforce these desires, make a list of all the positive aspects of eating right and working out, and post it so it's the first thing you see each morning. This list—the answer to this question—will give you passion-filled direction. For example, let's say you're following Body Fuel to improve the quality of your life. Once you know that and believe it, then your mind-set begins to change from "Am I going to eat healthfully today?" to "What am I going to eat today to improve the quality of my life?" Good nutrition thus becomes integrated into your life and lifestyle.

Military trainees know how to direct their passion into their mission. They're able to harness their mental and emotional power into what they've got to accomplish, whether that's completing a grueling training course or winning a battle. Translated to you and your fitness efforts, this means fortifying your mind with a can-do attitude. One powerful way to accomplish this is to have some personal affirmations ready to play and replay in your head. For example, replace "I can't stick to a good diet" with "I love feeding my body with quality food." Or replace "I don't feel like working out today" with "I will feel fantastic after I work out today."

Why would you ever tell yourself what you don't want to do? When the mind talks, the body listens. Not allowing negative self-talk or put-downs to enter your mind requires that you carefully listen to your mind chatter, booting out derogatory thoughts and allowing more enabling ones to take their place. At the end of every workout or every nutrition-filled day, identify something you did well. Let it run through your mind, imprint it on your brain, and celebrate that bit of success.

Remember, too, actions speak louder than words. All the positive thinking and talking in the world won't make you leaner, faster, stronger, or healthier. Consistent action, fortified by perseverance in healthful diet and exercise habits, is an inescapable ingredient of success.

When I train people, I constantly remind them that with each day of training, they make a choice to take a step toward completing their mission, remain the same, or take a step back. The same goes for you: each day you make a choice to stay on the plan or not, but that's your choice.

It helps to establish a specific mission for yourself each day before you begin the day. For example, tell yourself: "Today, I'm going to have a perfectly clean day of nutrition. No screw-ups!" Remind yourself of your mission for that day throughout the day.

You're in it for the long haul, so you must constantly review your mission, evaluate your own progress, acknowledge your successes and failures, and remain focused on moving forward. When you stay committed to your mission, it builds your passion—and your confidence—on a daily basis.

People are also passionate about activities they love. That's why I believe that you should make nutrition and exercise fun. I know what you're thinking: "Dieting, fun? Sweating, fun? Are you out of your mind?"

Hear me out. You can make these things more enjoyable. Swap tips and recipes with friends who are on Body Fuel. Put a dollar or some loose change in a jar every time you have a healthful week or do your workouts on schedule. Watch the loot pile up over a month, then spend it on something for yourself—but not a bunch of candy bars. Try a fun new fitness activity to complement your body-weight workouts. Maybe try kayaking, bicycling, or hiking, for example.

Also, I think you need to mentally frame up the outcomes you're looking for as fun: It's fun to wear skimpy clothes on your new hot body. It's fun to go shopping for new (smaller) clothes. It's fun to show off muscle definition at the beach. It's fun to have more energy and feel more vital. Not only are you looking for a great body and better health, you're also looking for a feeling—and that feeling is that it's fun to be in shape.

There's a great quote: "If the love of what you do exceeds the effort of doing it, success is inevitable." That's your career, that's play, that's parenting, that's being a good friend or partner or spouse, that's working out and eating healthfully. Once you really love what you're doing and have fun by doing it, you'll immediately start feeling better. Your energy levels will skyrocket. Your performance in all aspects of your life will increase as well. You'll be able to do a lot more with much less effort and energy.

Having passion is always best. You're going to live a better, more fulfilling life, with a smile on your face, projecting positivity.

I tell people this all the time: in order to transform your physique, you have to change your mind-set and your way of life.

Have the determination and passion that you're going to succeed. Take the responsibility to eat a healthful diet, exercise, and change your way of living.

People who do this with passion and direction amaze themselves at what they're capable of achieving.

Start amazing yourself today.

Acknowledgments

There are very few things worth mentioning that are accomplished alone. This book and its concept are the product of many talented and dedicated people. There are so many small and big pieces without which this work could not have been created. I want to thank you all.

My exceptional literary agent, Steve Ross, brought this team together and set the work in motion. My coauthor, Maggie Greenwood-Robinson, made the entire process feel almost effortless with her ability to ask the right questions, clearly express ideas, and organize information, and, most important, by simply being a great person to work with. Executive editor Marnie Cochran, at Ballantine Books, has put a lot of faith and trust in my team and guides these projects with great competence. Samantha Nomany and Sengfong Rozales have been massive contributors with their many hours of work, creating unique recipes that fit the guidelines of this diet.

Last and most important, I'd like to express my eternal appreciation to the true linchpin: the many users of my programs, who have provided me with invaluable support and feedback.

Appendix

MEAL PLANNING TEMPLATE

Here is a simple meal planner you can use for all three blocks of Body Fuel. In the weekly menu, simply fill in what you'll eat at each meal. In the shopping list, fill in the foods you'll need for each week of the Body Fuel plan.

MONDAY	TUESDAY
Breakfast: Protein: Fast Fuel: Other (Slow Fuel, Bonus Fuel, Condiment):	**Breakfast:** Protein: Fast Fuel: Other (Slow Fuel, Bonus Fuel, Condiment):
Snack: Protein: Fast Fuel: Other (Slow Fuel, Bonus Fuel, Condiment):	**Snack:** Protein: Fast Fuel: Other (Slow Fuel, Bonus Fuel, Condiment):
Lunch: Protein: Fast Fuel: Other (Slow Fuel, Bonus Fuel, Condiment):	**Lunch:** Protein: Fast Fuel: Other (Slow Fuel, Bonus Fuel, Condiment):
Snack: Protein: Slow Fuel: Other (Nuts, Seeds, or Bonus Fuel):	**Snack:** Protein: Slow Fuel: Other (Nuts, Seeds, or Bonus Fuel):
Dinner: Protein: Fast Fuel: Other (Slow Fuel, Bonus Fuel, Condiment):	**Dinner:** Protein: Fast Fuel: Other (Slow Fuel, Bonus Fuel, Condiment):

WEDNESDAY	THURSDAY
Breakfast: Protein: Fast Fuel: Other (Slow Fuel, Bonus Fuel, Condiment):	**Breakfast:** Protein: Fast Fuel: Other (Slow Fuel, Bonus Fuel, Condiment):
Snack: Protein: Fast Fuel: Other (Slow Fuel, Bonus Fuel, Condiment):	**Snack:** Protein: Fast Fuel: Other (Slow Fuel, Bonus Fuel, Condiment):
Lunch: Protein: Fast Fuel: Other (Slow Fuel, Bonus Fuel, Condiment):	**Lunch:** Protein: Fast Fuel: Other (Slow Fuel, Bonus Fuel, Condiment):
Snack: Protein: Slow Fuel: Other (Nuts, Seeds, or Bonus Fuel):	**Snack:** Protein: Slow Fuel: Other (Nuts, Seeds, or Bonus Fuel):
Dinner: Protein: Fast Fuel: Other (Slow Fuel, Bonus Fuel, Condiment):	**Dinner:** Protein: Fast Fuel: Other (Slow Fuel, Bonus Fuel, Condiment):

FRIDAY	SATURDAY
Breakfast: Protein: Fast Fuel: Other (Slow Fuel, Bonus Fuel, Condiment):	**Breakfast:** Protein: Fast Fuel: Other (Slow Fuel, Bonus Fuel, Condiment):
Snack: Protein: Fast Fuel: Other (Slow Fuel, Bonus Fuel, Condiment):	**Snack:** Protein: Fast Fuel: Other (Slow Fuel, Bonus Fuel, Condiment):
Lunch: Protein: Fast Fuel: Other (Slow Fuel, Bonus Fuel, Condiment):	**Lunch:** Protein: Fast Fuel: Other (Slow Fuel, Bonus Fuel, Condiment):
Snack: Protein: Slow Fuel: Other (Nuts, Seeds, or Bonus Fuel):	**Snack:** Protein: Slow Fuel: Other (Nuts, Seeds, or Bonus Fuel):
Dinner: Protein: Fast Fuel: Other (Slow Fuel, Bonus Fuel, Condiment):	**Dinner:** Protein: Fast Fuel: Other (Slow Fuel, Bonus Fuel, Condiment):

SUNDAY	Produce:
Breakfast:	Vegetables
Protein:	Fruits
Fast Fuel:	
Other (Slow Fuel, Bonus Fuel, Condiment):	**Proteins:**
	Meats and Poultry
Snack:	Seafood
Protein:	Eggs and Meat Alternatives
Fast Fuel:	
Other (Slow Fuel, Bonus Fuel, Condiment):	**Cereals, Grains, and Bread**
Lunch:	**Frozen Foods**
Protein:	
Fast Fuel:	**Canned Goods**
Other (Slow Fuel, Bonus Fuel, Condiment):	**Oils and Vinegar**
Snack:	
Protein:	**Spices**
Slow Fuel:	
Other (Nuts, Seeds, or Bonus Fuel):	**Condiments and Sweetening Agents**
Dinner:	**Beverages**
Protein:	**Miscellaneous**
Fast Fuel:	
Other (Slow Fuel, Bonus Fuel, Condiment):	

MONDAY	TUESDAY
Breakfast: Protein: Fast Fuel: Other (Slow Fuel, Bonus Fuel, Condiment):	**Breakfast:** Protein: Fast Fuel: Other (Slow Fuel, Bonus Fuel, Condiment):
Snack: Protein: Fast Fuel: Other (Slow Fuel, Bonus Fuel, Condiment):	**Snack:** Protein: Fast Fuel: Other (Slow Fuel, Bonus Fuel, Condiment):
Lunch: Protein: Fast Fuel: Other (Slow Fuel, Bonus Fuel, Condiment):	**Lunch:** Protein: Fast Fuel: Other (Slow Fuel, Bonus Fuel, Condiment):
Snack: Protein: Slow Fuel: Other (Nuts, Seeds, or Bonus Fuel):	**Snack:** Protein: Slow Fuel: Other (Nuts, Seeds, or Bonus Fuel):
Dinner: Protein: Fast Fuel: Other (Slow Fuel, Bonus Fuel, Condiment):	**Dinner:** Protein: Fast Fuel: Other (Slow Fuel, Bonus Fuel, Condiment):

WEDNESDAY	THURSDAY
Breakfast: Protein: Fast Fuel: Other (Slow Fuel, Bonus Fuel, Condiment):	**Breakfast:** Protein: Fast Fuel: Other (Slow Fuel, Bonus Fuel, Condiment):
Snack: Protein: Fast Fuel: Other (Slow Fuel, Bonus Fuel, Condiment):	**Snack:** Protein: Fast Fuel: Other (Slow Fuel, Bonus Fuel, Condiment):
Lunch: Protein: Fast Fuel: Other (Slow Fuel, Bonus Fuel, Condiment):	**Lunch:** Protein: Fast Fuel: Other (Slow Fuel, Bonus Fuel, Condiment):
Snack: Protein: Slow Fuel: Other (Nuts, Seeds, or Bonus Fuel):	**Snack:** Protein: Slow Fuel: Other (Nuts, Seeds, or Bonus Fuel):
Dinner: Protein: Fast Fuel: Other (Slow Fuel, Bonus Fuel, Condiment):	**Dinner:** Protein: Fast Fuel: Other (Slow Fuel, Bonus Fuel, Condiment):

FRIDAY	SATURDAY
Breakfast: Protein: Fast Fuel: Other (Slow Fuel, Bonus Fuel, Condiment):	**Breakfast:** Protein: Fast Fuel: Other (Slow Fuel, Bonus Fuel, Condiment):
Snack: Protein: Fast Fuel: Other (Slow Fuel, Bonus Fuel, Condiment):	**Snack:** Protein: Fast Fuel: Other (Slow Fuel, Bonus Fuel, Condiment):
Lunch: Protein: Fast Fuel: Other (Slow Fuel, Bonus Fuel, Condiment):	**Lunch:** Protein: Fast Fuel: Other (Slow Fuel, Bonus Fuel, Condiment):
Snack: Protein: Slow Fuel: Other (Nuts, Seeds, or Bonus Fuel):	**Snack:** Protein: Slow Fuel: Other (Nuts, Seeds, or Bonus Fuel):
Dinner: Protein: Fast Fuel: Other (Slow Fuel, Bonus Fuel, Condiment):	**Dinner:** Protein: Fast Fuel: Other (Slow Fuel, Bonus Fuel, Condiment):

SUNDAY

Breakfast:

Protein:

Fast Fuel:

Other (Slow Fuel, Bonus Fuel, Condiment):

Snack:

Protein:

Fast Fuel:

Other (Slow Fuel, Bonus Fuel, Condiment):

Lunch:

Protein:

Fast Fuel:

Other (Slow Fuel, Bonus Fuel, Condiment):

Snack:

Protein:

Slow Fuel:

Other (Nuts, Seeds, or Bonus Fuel):

Dinner:

Protein:

Fast Fuel:

Other (Slow Fuel, Bonus Fuel, Condiment):

Produce:

Vegetables

Fruits

Proteins:

Meats and Poultry

Seafood

Eggs and Meat Alternatives

Cereals, Grains, and Bread

Frozen Foods

Canned Goods

Oils and Vinegar

Spices

Condiments and Sweetening Agents

Beverages

Miscellaneous

MONDAY	TUESDAY
Breakfast: Protein: Fast Fuel: Other (Slow Fuel, Bonus Fuel, Condiment):	**Breakfast:** Protein: Fast Fuel: Other (Slow Fuel, Bonus Fuel, Condiment):
Snack: Protein: Fast Fuel: Other (If not eaten at breakfast):	**Snack:** Protein: Fast Fuel: Other (If not eaten at breakfast):
Lunch: Protein: Fast Fuel: Other (Slow Fuel, Bonus Fuel, Condiment):	**Lunch:** Protein: Fast Fuel: Other (Slow Fuel, Bonus Fuel, Condiment):
Snack: Protein: Slow Fuel: Other (Nuts, Seeds, or Bonus Fuel):	**Snack:** Protein: Slow Fuel: Other (Nuts, Seeds, or Bonus Fuel):
Dinner: Protein: Fast Fuel: Other (Slow Fuel, Bonus Fuel, Condiment):	**Dinner:** Protein: Fast Fuel: Other (Slow Fuel, Bonus Fuel, Condiment):

WEDNESDAY	THURSDAY
Breakfast: Protein: Fast Fuel: Other (Slow Fuel, Bonus Fuel, Condiment):	**Breakfast:** Protein: Fast Fuel: Other (Slow Fuel, Bonus Fuel, Condiment):
Snack: Protein: Fast Fuel: Other (If not eaten at breakfast):	**Snack:** Protein: Fast Fuel: Other (If not eaten at breakfast):
Lunch: Protein: Fast Fuel: Other (Slow Fuel, Bonus Fuel, Condiment):	**Lunch:** Protein: Fast Fuel: Other (Slow Fuel, Bonus Fuel, Condiment):
Snack: Protein: Slow Fuel: Other (Nuts, Seeds, or Bonus Fuel):	**Snack:** Protein: Slow Fuel: Other (Nuts, Seeds, or Bonus Fuel):
Dinner: Protein: Fast Fuel: Other (Slow Fuel, Bonus Fuel, Condiment):	**Dinner:** Protein: Fast Fuel: Other (Slow Fuel, Bonus Fuel, Condiment):

FRIDAY	SATURDAY
Breakfast: Protein: Fast Fuel: Other (Slow Fuel, Bonus Fuel, Condiment):	**Breakfast:** Protein: Fast Fuel: Other (Slow Fuel, Bonus Fuel, Condiment):
Snack: Protein: Fast Fuel: Other (If not eaten at breakfast):	**Snack:** Protein: Fast Fuel: Other (If not eaten at breakfast):
Lunch: Protein: Fast Fuel: Other (Slow Fuel, Bonus Fuel, Condiment):	**Lunch:** Protein: Fast Fuel: Other (Slow Fuel, Bonus Fuel, Condiment):
Snack: Protein: Slow Fuel: Other (Nuts, Seeds, or Bonus Fuel):	**Snack:** Protein: Slow Fuel: Other (Nuts, Seeds, or Bonus Fuel):
Dinner: Protein: Fast Fuel: Other (Slow Fuel, Bonus Fuel, Condiment):	**Dinner:** Protein: Fast Fuel: Other (Slow Fuel, Bonus Fuel, Condiment):

SUNDAY

Breakfast:

Protein:

Fast Fuel:

Other (Slow Fuel, Bonus Fuel, Condiment):

Snack:

Protein:

Fast Fuel:

Other (If not eaten at breakfast):

Lunch:

Protein:

Fast Fuel:

Other (Slow Fuel, Bonus Fuel, Condiment):

Snack:

Protein:

Slow Fuel:

Other (Nuts, Seeds, or Bonus Fuel):

Dinner:

Protein:

Fast Fuel:

Other (Slow Fuel, Bonus Fuel, Condiment):

Produce:

Vegetables

Fruits

Proteins:

Meats and Poultry

Seafood

Eggs and Meat Alternatives

Cereals, Grains, and Bread

Frozen Foods

Canned Goods

Oils and Vinegar

Spices

Condiments and Sweetening Agents

Beverages

Miscellaneous

Bibliography

PART 1: MASTER THE SCIENCE OF A FIRM, FAT-FREE BODY

Chapter 2: The Other Body Fuels: Protein and Fat

Bazzano, L. A., et al. 2014. Effects of low-carbohydrate and low-fat diets: a randomized trial. *Annals of Internal Medicine* 161:309–318.

Bendtsen, L. Q., et al. 2013. Effect of dairy proteins on appetite, energy expenditure, body weight, and composition: a review of the evidence from controlled clinical trials. *Advances in Nutrition* 4:418–438.

Boschmann, M., et al. 2003. Water-induced thermogenesis. *Journal of Clinical Endocrinology and Metabolism* 88:6015–6019.

Halton, T. L., and F. B. Hu. 2004. The effects of high protein diets on thermogenesis, satiety and weight loss: a critical review. *Journal of the American College of Nutrition* 23:373–385.

Hämäläinen, E. K., et al. 1983. Decrease of serum total and free testosterone during a low-fat high-fibre diet. *Journal of Steroid Biochemistry* 18:369–370.

Johnstone, A. M., et al. 2012. Safety and efficacy of high-protein diets for weight loss. *Proceedings of the Nutrition Society* 71:339–349.

Judelson, D. A., et al. 2008. Effect of hydration state on resistance exercise-induced endocrine markers of anabolism, catabolism, and metabolism. *Journal of Applied Physiology* 105:816–824.

Layman, D. K., and D. A. Walker. 2006. Potential importance of leucine in treatment of obesity and the metabolic syndrome. *Journal of Nutrition* 136:319S–323S.

Sawka, M. N., et al. 2007. Position stand on exercise and fluid replacement. *Medicine and Science in Sports and Exercise* 39:377–390.

Siri-Tarino, P. W., et al. 2010. Saturated fat, carbohydrate, and cardiovascular disease. *American Journal of Clinical Nutrition* 91:502–509.

Chapter 3: Calorie Cycling

Davoodi, S. H., et al. 2014. Calorie shifting diet versus calorie restriction diet: a comparative clinical trial study. *International Journal of Preventive Medicine* 5:447–456.

Farshchi, H. R., et al. 2005. Beneficial metabolic effects of regular meal frequency on dietary thermogenesis, insulin sensitivity, and fasting lipid profiles in healthy obese women. *American Journal of Clinical Nutrition* 81:16–24.

Jenkins, D. J., et al. 1989. Nibbling versus gorging: metabolic advantages of increased meal frequency. *New England Journal of Medicine* 321:929–934.

Kohlstadt, I. 2008. Optimizing metabolism: obesity-exacerbating conditions (report). *Townsend Report*, June 1.

PART 2: REAL FUEL

Chapter 4: What to Eat: The Magnificent 7

Golding, J., et al. 2013. Dietary predictors of maternal prenatal blood mercury levels in the ALSPAC birth cohort study. *Environmental Health Perspectives* 121:1214–1218.

McAfee, A. J., et al. 2011. Red meat from animals offered a grass diet increases plasma and platelet n-3 PUFA in healthy consumers. *British Journal of Nutrition* 105:80–89.

Morganstern, I., et al. 2011. Regulation of drug and palatable food overconsumption by similar peptide systems. *Current Drug Abuse Reviews* 4:163–173.

Ostman, E. M., et al. 2001. Inconsistency between glycemic and insulinemic responses to regular and fermented milk products. *American Journal of Clinical Nutrition* 74:96–100.

Roosevelt, M. 2006. The grass-fed revolution. Beef raised wholly on pasture, rather than grain-fed in feedlots, may be better for your health—and for the planet. *Time*, June 12, 76–78.

Vander Wal, J. S., et al. 2005. Short-term effect of eggs on satiety in overweight and obese subjects. *Journal of the American College of Nutrition* 24:510–515.

Chapter 6: Zero Week—Fall In!

Bes Rastrollo, M., et al. 2008. Prospective study of dietary energy density and weight gain in women. *American Journal of Clinical Nutrition* 88:769–777.

Hollis, J. F., et al. 2008. Weight loss during the intensive intervention phase of the weight-loss maintenance trial. *American Journal of Preventive Medicine* 35:118–126.

Rolls, B. J., et al. 2004. Salad and satiety: energy density and portion size of a first-course salad affect energy intake at lunch. *Journal of the American Dietetic Association* 104:1570–1576.

Wolf, A., et al. 2008. A short history of beverages and how our body treats them. *Obesity Reviews* 9:151–164.

PART 3: POWER UP

Chapter 10: Fuel Tools: Body Fuel Supplements

Abou-Samra, R., et al. 2011. Effect of different protein sources on satiation and short-term satiety when consumed as a starter. *Nutrition Journal* 10:139.

Baer, D. J., et al. 2011. Whey protein but not soy protein supplementation alters body weight and composition in free-living overweight and obese adults. *Journal of Nutrition* 141:1489–1494.

Fortmann, S. P., et al. 2013. Vitamin and mineral supplements in the primary prevention of cardiovascular disease and cancer: an updated systematic evidence review for the U.S. Preventive Services Task Force. *Annals of Internal Medicine* 159:824–834.

PART 4: THE BODY FUEL WORKOUT

Chapter 11: A Quicker System for Faster Results

Schuenke, M. D., et al. 2002. Effect of an acute period of resistance exercise on excess post-exercise oxygen consumption: implications for body mass management. *European Journal of Applied Physiology* 86:411–417.

Chapter 13: Body Fuel in the Real World

Klem, M. L., et al. 2000. Does weight loss maintenance become easier over time? *Obesity Research* 8:438–444.

McGuire, M. T., et al. 1999. Behavioral strategies of individuals who have maintained long-term weight losses. *Obesity Research* 7:334–341.

Wing, R. R., and J. O. Hill. 2001. Successful weight loss maintenance. *Annual Review of Nutrition* 21:323–341.

Wyatt, H. R., et al. 2002. Long-term weight loss and breakfast in subjects in the National Weight Control Registry. *Obesity Research* 10:78–82.

About the Authors

MARK LAUREN spent fifteen years in the Special Operations community as an operator and physical training specialist. He is the author of the internationally popular body-weight bibles *You Are Your Own Gym* and *Body by You* and a sought-after personal trainer to civilian men and women of all fitness levels. He is a triathlete and former Thai boxing champion living in Phuket, Thailand.

MarkLauren.com
Facebook.com/bodyweight
@yourowngym

MAGGIE GREENWOOD-ROBINSON is a *New York Times* bestselling collaborator who specializes in health and fitness. She lives in Dallas, Texas.